When Abortion Is Not an Option

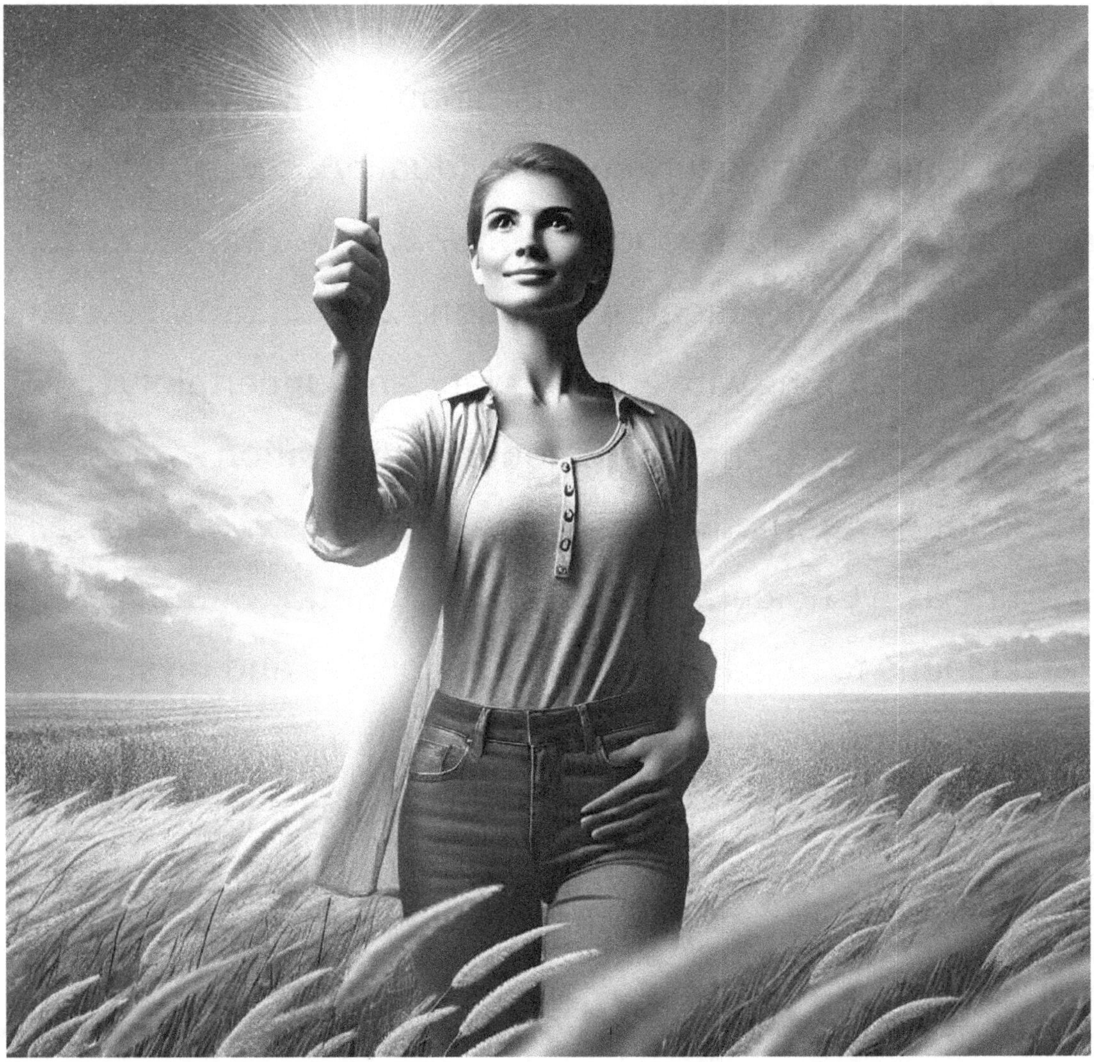

A Guide for Women

Robert Anderson Love Wins

http://RobertAndersonLoveWins.com

Table of Contents

Part I: Understanding the Context 8

1. The Decision to Continue the Pregnancy 8

Personal, Cultural, and Religious Influences 8

Medical Reasons for Continuing Pregnancy.............................. 10

Acknowledging Complexity and Individuality 11

2. Navigating Emotional Responses... 13

Acknowledging and Validating Emotions 13

Strategies for Coping with Fear, Anxiety, and Uncertainty 14

Recognizing Growth Through Emotional Navigation 17

Part II: Exploring Alternatives 18

3. Parenting as a Choice 18

What It Means to Be a Parent: Responsibilities and Joys............. 18

Accessing Parental Support Networks 20

Parenting Classes and Educational Resources 21

Final Thoughts on Parenting as a Choice 23

4. Understanding Adoption 24

Types of Adoption: Open, Closed, and Semi-Open 25

The Adoption Process: Steps, Resources, and Emotional
Considerations 27

Stories from Birth Mothers: Perspectives on Adoption 29

Final Thoughts on Adoption 30

5. Exploring Foster Care as an Option 31

What is Foster Care? 31

The Process of Placing a Child in Foster Care 32

Support for Mothers Considering Foster Care 33

Final Thoughts on Foster Care as an Option 35

Part III: Building a Support System 36

6. Turning to Family and Friends 36

How to Share Your Decision and Ask for Help 36

Navigating Supportive and Unsupportive Reactions 38

Practical Tips for Strengthening Your Support Network 39

Final Thoughts on Turning to Family and Friends 40

7. Counseling and Emotional Support 41

Finding Professional Counseling Services 41

Joining Support Groups for Pregnant Women 43

The Role of Peer Networks in Providing Emotional Strength 44

Final Thoughts on Counseling and Emotional Support 46

8.   Pregnancy Resource Centers 47

Shelters, Food Banks, and Local Organizations 48

Maximizing the Benefits of Community Resources 50

Final Thoughts on Community Resources for Women 51

Part IV: Practical Considerations 52

9. Financial Planning and Support 52

Budgeting for a Baby: Essentials and Tips 52

Government Assistance Programs (WIC, TANF, Medicaid) 54

Childcare Options and Subsidies 55

Final Thoughts on Financial Planning and Support 57

10.   Accessing Prenatal Care: Clinics, Hospitals, and Low-Cost Options 58

Maternal Health: Physical and Emotional Well-Being 59

Postnatal Care for Mother and Baby 61

Final Thoughts on Healthcare During Pregnancy 63

11.   Custody and Parental Responsibilities 65

Child Support and Financial Obligations 66

Resources for Legal Assistance 67

Tips for Navigating Legal Processes 68

Final Thoughts on Understanding Your Legal Rights 69

Part V: Emotional and Psychological Support 70

12. Coping with Stress and Anxiety 70

Mindfulness Practices and Breathing Exercises 70

Journaling Prompts for Emotional Clarity 71

Self-Care Strategies for Mental Health 72

13. Affirmations and Positive Thinking 75

Cultivating a Supportive Inner Dialogue 75

Examples of Affirmations for Strength and Resilience 76

Tips for Using Affirmations Effectively 78

Part VI: Stories and Inspiration 80

14. Personal Testimonials 80

Stories from Women Who Chose Parenting 80

Perspectives from Birth Mothers Who Chose Adoption 81

Stories of Resilience from Women Who Found Support 81

Final Thoughts on Personal Testimonials 82

Part VII: Resources and Tools 83

15. Recommended Reading and Media 83

Books on Parenting, Adoption, and Emotional Healing.............. 83

Articles Offering Practical Advice and Emotional Support 85

How to Use These Resources 87

16. Hotlines for Counseling and Pregnancy Support 89

Websites for Local and National Resources 90

Organizations Offering Free or Low-Cost Services 92

Part VIII: Creating a Vision for the Future 95

17. Setting Personal Goals 95

Envisioning Life After Pregnancy 95

Tools for Building a Fulfilling Future.. 97

Tips for Staying Motivated.. 99

18. Empowerment and Resilience 101

Stories of Women Who Thrived Despite Challenges................. 101

Building Confidence and Finding Your Strength 102

Resilience Strategies for Building a Fulfilling Life 104

Part IX: Workshops and Learning Opportunities 106

19. Parenting and Personal Development Classes...................... 106

Workshops on Parenting Skills and Emotional Intelligence....... 106

Financial Literacy and Budgeting Programs 108

Personal Growth and Development Opportunities 109

Part X: Frequently Asked Questions 113

20. Common Concerns and Answers 113

Pregnancy FAQs: Health, Support, and Logistics 113

Parenting FAQs: Planning for the First Year 115

Adoption FAQs: Understanding the Process and Emotions....... 117

Closing Section: Words of Encouragement 119

21. A Message of Hope and Strength 119

Remembering You Are Not Alone 119

Finding Your Path Forward with Confidence............................ 121

Disclaimer 124

Ending Letter of Encouragement 125

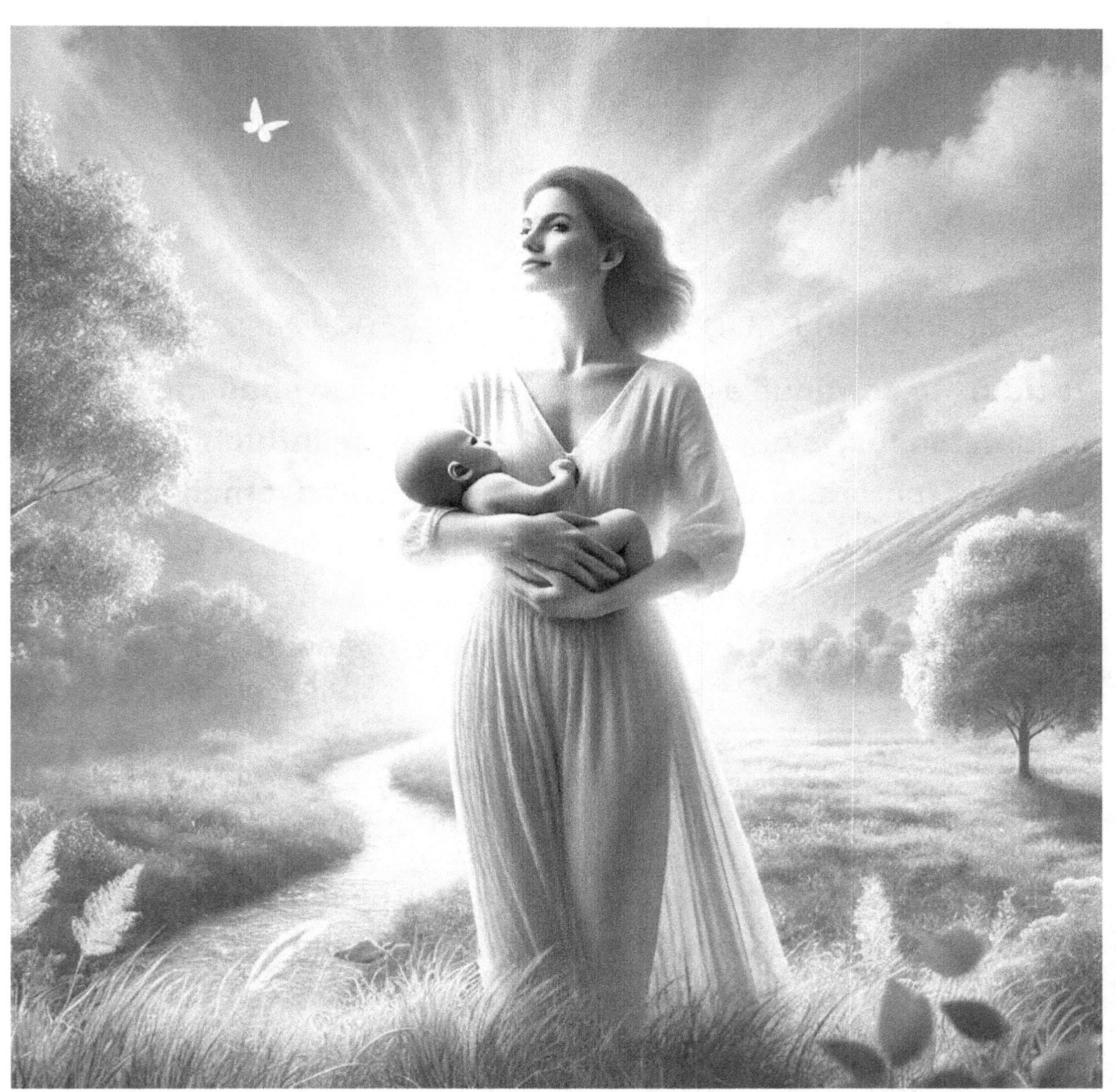

Part I: Understanding the Context

1. The Decision to Continue the Pregnancy

Deciding to continue a pregnancy, especially in challenging circumstances, is deeply personal and can be influenced by a variety of factors. This decision often reflects a woman's values, beliefs, and unique life situation. Whether motivated by cultural, religious, personal, or medical reasons, it's a choice that deserves understanding, support, and compassion.

Personal, Cultural, and Religious Influences

1. **Personal Values and Beliefs**
   Many women choose to continue a pregnancy based on deeply held personal convictions about life and its sanctity. These values might stem from a sense of moral duty, a commitment to nurturing, or a belief in the intrinsic potential of every life.

   - **Some may feel that continuing the pregnancy aligns with their personal definition of integrity or responsibility.**

   - **Others might view the challenge as an opportunity for growth, strength, or transformation.**

2. **Cultural Expectations**
   Cultural norms and traditions can play a significant role in shaping a woman's decision.

   - In some cultures, motherhood is highly revered, and continuing a pregnancy may be seen as fulfilling a vital role within the community or family.

   - Women may also feel influenced by cultural stigmas surrounding abortion, choosing to continue the pregnancy to honor societal expectations or family traditions.

3. **Religious Convictions**
   Religious beliefs are often a guiding force in such decisions. Many faiths teach that life begins at conception and that every life is sacred, emphasizing the importance of nurturing and protecting the unborn.

   - A woman may feel a spiritual responsibility to continue the pregnancy, trusting in divine guidance to help her navigate the challenges ahead.

   - Support from religious communities often reinforces this choice, providing comfort and practical assistance grounded in shared beliefs.

4. **Influence of Family and Partners**
   Loved ones, including family members and partners, may express strong opinions or provide support that affects the decision.

- Positive encouragement from trusted individuals can bolster a woman's confidence in continuing the pregnancy.

- Open communication with loved ones can help clarify priorities and build a supportive foundation for the journey ahead.

Medical Reasons for Continuing Pregnancy

1. **Health and Safety Considerations**
   For some women, medical factors make abortion a less viable or inadvisable option.

   - Pre-existing health conditions, such as heart disease or blood clotting disorders, may make certain medical procedures more risky.

   - If a pregnancy is further along, the risks associated with termination may outweigh the potential benefits, prompting a decision to continue.

2. **Fetal Viability and Development**
   Advances in medical technology allow for greater understanding of fetal development.

   - Some women may decide to continue a pregnancy after learning that the fetus is healthy and thriving, despite initial uncertainties.

- Ultrasounds, genetic testing, and other prenatal diagnostics can provide reassurance that the baby has a strong chance of survival and health.

3. **Unexpected Maternal Health Improvements**
   Occasionally, conditions initially thought to complicate a pregnancy, such as hyperemesis gravidarum or gestational diabetes, may improve with proper treatment.

   - When medical management is effective, women may find continuing the pregnancy more feasible than initially anticipated.

4. **Desire to Protect Future Fertility**
   Some women may choose to continue a pregnancy out of concern for their long-term reproductive health.

   - Certain medical procedures or complications from termination could affect future fertility, influencing the decision to proceed with the current pregnancy.

Acknowledging Complexity and Individuality

Every woman's situation is unique, and the decision to continue a pregnancy reflects a complex interplay of personal values, external influences, and medical realities. It is important to approach this decision with sensitivity and empathy, recognizing the strength it takes to navigate such a significant choice.

By understanding the personal, cultural, religious, and medical factors that inform this decision, women can feel empowered to make choices that honor their beliefs, protect their health, and align with their vision for the future. With access to support and resources, this decision can become a pathway to strength, resilience, and personal growth.

Deciding to continue a pregnancy, especially in unexpected or challenging circumstances, can evoke a wide range of emotions. It's natural to feel fear, anxiety, doubt, or even moments of hope and excitement. These emotions are valid and reflect the depth of the situation. Recognizing and managing these feelings is a vital part of navigating this journey with strength and clarity.

Acknowledging and Validating Emotions

1. **Understanding Emotional Complexity**

   - **Women in this situation often experience a blend of conflicting emotions, including fear, guilt, confusion, hope, and even acceptance.**

   - **It's essential to understand that feeling overwhelmed or unsure doesn't mean you're incapable of handling the situation. It means you're processing a significant life event.**

2. **Allowing Yourself to Feel Without Judgment**

   - **It's okay to feel scared, sad, or uncertain. These emotions don't make you weak—they make you human.**

   - **Avoid suppressing emotions; instead, allow yourself to acknowledge them. Journaling, speaking with a trusted confidant, or even quietly reflecting can help validate your feelings.**

3. **Recognizing the Role of External Pressures**

   - External opinions from family, friends, or society may amplify emotional responses. Understanding the difference between your feelings and others' expectations is key to processing emotions authentically.

   - Trust your internal compass. Your feelings are valid regardless of external judgments.

4. **Seeking Compassion and Support**

   - Share your emotions with people who will listen without judgment. Whether it's a close friend, family member, or counselor, finding a safe space to express yourself can be profoundly healing.

Strategies for Coping with Fear, Anxiety, and Uncertainty

1. **Focus on What You Can Control**

   - Fear and anxiety often stem from focusing on uncertainties or worst-case scenarios. Shift your energy to what you can control, such as seeking resources, planning for the future, and caring for your health.

   - Make a list of small, actionable steps you can take daily. Breaking larger tasks into manageable pieces can reduce feelings of overwhelm.

○

2. Practice Mindfulness and Stress Management

- ○ **Incorporate calming practices into your routine, such as mindfulness meditation, deep breathing exercises, or yoga. These activities help center your thoughts and bring your focus to the present moment.**

- ○ **Spend time in nature, even for short walks. Natural surroundings can have a calming effect and help reset your perspective.**

3. Connect with Support Networks

- ○ **Join support groups or forums for women experiencing similar situations. Knowing that you're not alone can alleviate feelings of isolation and offer valuable insights.**

- ○ **Reach out to local pregnancy centers, counselors, or social workers who specialize in providing emotional and practical support.**

4. Reframe Negative Thoughts

- ○ **Challenge catastrophic thinking. For example, if you think, *"I won't be able to handle this,"* replace it with, *"I may face challenges, but I can seek help and find solutions."***

- ○ **Remind yourself that you're capable of growth and resilience, even in difficult situations. Affirmations like**

"I am stronger than I realize" can help reframe negative thought patterns.

5. Maintain Self-Care Practices

- Prioritize basic self-care, including eating well, staying hydrated, and getting enough rest. A healthy body supports a balanced mind.

- Schedule moments of joy and relaxation, even if it's something small like reading, listening to music, or enjoying a favorite hobby.

6. Seek Professional Help When Needed

- If fear or anxiety becomes overwhelming, consider speaking with a licensed counselor or therapist. They can provide coping strategies tailored to your needs and offer a space for healing.

- Therapy can also help address feelings of guilt, shame, or inadequacy, replacing them with a sense of empowerment and self-compassion.

Processing emotional responses is not about eliminating difficult feelings but learning how to navigate them with grace and resilience. Each step you take to acknowledge your emotions and manage them positively strengthens your ability to face challenges with courage.

Remember, your feelings are valid, and seeking support is a sign of strength, not weakness. With the right tools and a compassionate support network, you can navigate fear, anxiety, and uncertainty to find clarity, hope, and confidence in your journey ahead.

3. Parenting as a Choice

Parenting is a profound and life-changing decision, marked by responsibilities, challenges, and immeasurable joys. For women who decide to embrace parenting, understanding what it entails and accessing the right support can make the journey enriching and rewarding. This chapter explores the meaning of parenthood, provides guidance on finding support networks, and highlights resources to help you grow into this important role.

What It Means to Be a Parent: Responsibilities and Joys

1. The Responsibilities of Parenthood

- **Emotional Nurturing: Parenting involves creating a safe, loving environment where your child can grow emotionally and develop confidence. This includes being present, patient, and responsive to their needs.**

- **Physical Care: Providing for your child's basic needs such as food, shelter, clothing, and healthcare is a fundamental aspect of parenthood.**

- **Guidance and Discipline: Teaching children values, life skills, and appropriate behaviors equips them to navigate the world. This includes setting boundaries and serving as a role model.**

- Financial Responsibility: Budgeting for your child's needs, from diapers to education, is part of the ongoing commitment to their well-being.

2. The Joys of Parenthood

- Unconditional Love: Many parents describe an indescribable bond that forms with their child, bringing profound feelings of love and purpose.

- Watching Growth and Milestones: Witnessing your child's first smile, first steps, and evolving personality is a source of pride and happiness.

- Creating a Legacy: Parenting allows you to pass on traditions, values, and wisdom, contributing to the shaping of a new generation.

- Personal Growth: While parenting challenges you, it also fosters resilience, patience, and a deeper sense of gratitude for life's small moments.

3. Balancing Challenges with Rewards

- It's natural to feel overwhelmed at times, especially as you adapt to new responsibilities. Remember that the joys of parenting often emerge from the effort and dedication you invest.

- Celebrating small victories—like soothing a crying baby or teaching your child a new skill—helps maintain a positive perspective.

1. Family and Friends

- o **Trusted Loved Ones: Relying on close family members or friends can provide emotional support and practical help, such as babysitting, advice, or simply someone to talk to.**

- o **Building a "Village": Surrounding yourself with supportive individuals fosters a network that can uplift you during challenging times.**

2. Community Support Groups

- o **Parenting Support Groups: Many local and online groups bring parents together to share experiences, offer advice, and create a sense of belonging.**

- o **Faith-Based Communities: Churches, temples, and other spiritual organizations often have programs for parents, such as childcare, counseling, or educational workshops.**

3. Local Resources

- o **Nonprofit Organizations: Many nonprofits offer assistance to new parents, including parenting classes, material supplies, and emotional support.**

- o **Government Programs: Look into programs like Women, Infants, and Children (WIC) and Medicaid for financial and healthcare assistance.**

4. **Online Networks**

   - ○ **Platforms like Facebook and parenting forums provide a space to connect with other parents, ask questions, and find encouragement from those who understand your journey.**

---

1. **Why Parenting Education Matters**

   - ○ **Parenting is a skill that grows over time. Attending classes or using educational resources can prepare you for challenges and give you tools to respond effectively to your child's needs.**

2. **Available Classes**

   - ○ **Prenatal and Postnatal Classes: Focused on the early stages of parenting, these classes cover topics like newborn care, breastfeeding, and postpartum recovery.**

   - ○ **Parenting Skills Workshops: Covering topics such as positive discipline, communication strategies, and developmental milestones, these workshops help parents feel more confident and equipped.**

   - ○ **Specialized Classes: Classes on topics like single parenting, co-parenting after separation, or raising** children with special needs provide tailored advice for unique situations.

3. **Where to Find Classes**

   - **Hospitals and Clinics:** Many hospitals offer prenatal and parenting classes as part of their maternity services.

   - **Community Centers:** Local community centers often host free or low-cost workshops for parents.

   - **Online Courses:** Websites like BabyCenter, Bright Horizons, and local nonprofit organizations offer virtual classes you can access from home.

4. **Books and Media**

   - **Books:** Recommended titles include *What to Expect When You're Expecting* by Heidi Murkoff and *Parenting with Love and Logic* by Charles Fay and Foster Cline.

   - **Podcasts and Videos:** Platforms like YouTube and Spotify feature parenting podcasts and instructional videos on topics ranging from baby care to teen parenting.

Parenthood is a journey of growth, love, and commitment. While it comes with significant responsibilities, it also offers unparalleled rewards, including the opportunity to shape a new life and create lasting bonds.

By surrounding yourself with supportive networks and seeking out educational resources, you can build a strong foundation for your parenting journey. Remember, no parent is perfect, but with intention, care, and persistence, you can provide a loving and nurturing environment where both you and your child can thrive.

4. Understanding Adoption

Adoption is a deeply personal and impactful choice for women facing pregnancy when parenting is not an option. It offers the opportunity to provide a child with a loving home while giving the birth mother a path forward that aligns with her circumstances. Understanding the types of adoption, the steps involved in the process, and the emotional considerations can empower women to make informed and compassionate decisions.

1. Open Adoption

- **Definition: Open adoption involves ongoing contact between the birth mother, adoptive parents, and, in some cases, the child. The level of communication is agreed upon by both parties.**
- **Benefits:**
  - **Allows the birth mother to stay connected with the child and observe their growth.**
  - **Creates transparency, reducing uncertainty and fostering trust.**
  - **Gives the child access to their biological history and identity.**
- **Challenges:**
  - **Requires clear boundaries and mutual respect.**
  - **Communication must be carefully managed to avoid misunderstandings.**

2. Closed Adoption

- **Definition: In a closed adoption, there is no contact between the birth mother and the adoptive family after the adoption is finalized. Records may be sealed, with limited or no access to identifying information.**

- Benefits:
    - Provides a clean emotional break for the birth mother.
    - Offers privacy for all parties involved.
- Challenges:
    - May leave the birth mother and child with unanswered questions.
    - Can create emotional distance that some may find difficult to reconcile later.

3. Semi-Open Adoption

- Definition: This option balances the characteristics of open and closed adoption. Communication between the birth mother and adoptive family is mediated through an agency or attorney.
- Benefits:
    - Provides limited contact while maintaining privacy.
    - Allows for updates about the child's well-being without direct interaction.
- Challenges:
    - The lack of direct communication may create ambiguity or unmet expectations.

1. Steps in the Adoption Process

- **Research and Decision-Making:**
    - **Explore different types of adoption to determine which option feels right for you.**
    - **Speak with adoption agencies or professionals to understand the specifics of each approach.**

- **Selecting an Adoption Agency or Facilitator:**
    - **Look for licensed, reputable organizations that align with your values.**
    - **Ask about services, such as counseling, financial assistance, and post-adoption support.**

- **Creating an Adoption Plan:**
    - **Work with your agency or attorney to outline preferences for the adoptive family, communication agreements, and other considerations.**

- **Matching with an Adoptive Family:**
    - **Review profiles of prospective adoptive families and participate in interviews if applicable.**
    - **Trust your instincts when selecting the right family for your child.**

- o **Legal Finalization:**
  - ▪ Ensure all legal requirements are met, including signing consent forms and attending necessary court proceedings.

2. **Resources for Birth Mothers**

- o **Adoption Agencies:** Organizations like Bethany Christian Services or American Adoptions provide comprehensive support throughout the process.
- o **Counseling Services:** Seek professional counseling to navigate the emotional complexities of adoption.
- o **Financial Assistance:** Some agencies or state programs offer financial support for medical expenses and other pregnancy-related costs.

3. **Emotional Considerations**

- o **Grief and Loss:** Placing a child for adoption can involve feelings of loss and sadness. Recognizing these emotions is essential for healing.
- o **Relief and Peace:** Many birth mothers feel a sense of relief knowing their child is placed in a loving home.
- o **Support Systems:** Surround yourself with understanding friends, family, or support groups who can offer encouragement and empathy.

    ○ **Ongoing Relationship Dynamics: If choosing open or semi-open adoption, prepare for evolving relationships with the adoptive family and child over time.**

---

1. **Finding Peace Through Open Adoption**
   "When I discovered I was pregnant, I was terrified. Parenting wasn't an option for me, but I couldn't imagine never knowing my child. Choosing open adoption gave me the chance to stay connected. I now receive updates and photos, and I know my child is happy. It's not always easy, but I feel peace knowing I made the right choice." – Sarah, **birth mother**

2. **Empowerment in Choosing Adoption**
   "Adoption was the hardest decision I've ever made, but it was also the most loving one. I chose a closed adoption because I needed space to heal and move forward. My agency provided amazing support, and I'm proud of the strength it took to make that decision." – Lisa, **birth mother**

3. **Building a Bridge with Semi-Open Adoption**
   "Semi-open adoption worked perfectly for me. I wanted to know my baby was cared for, but I didn't feel ready for direct communication. I receive letters and photos through the agency, and it gives me reassurance. Over time, I've started to feel proud of my choice." – Maria, **birth mother**

Adoption is a deeply personal decision that requires thought, courage, and compassion. Whether you choose open, closed, or semi-open adoption, each path offers the opportunity to provide your child with a loving family while honoring your own needs and circumstances.

By understanding the types of adoption, preparing for the process, and seeking the right support, you can make a choice that reflects love, integrity, and hope for the future. Adoption is not just a decision—it's a testament to your strength and your belief in what's best for your child.

5. Exploring Foster Care as an Option

Foster care is a temporary solution for mothers who may not feel prepared or able to care for their child immediately after birth. It provides a structured environment where children are cared for by trained families or institutions while mothers determine the best long-term plans for their child's future. Choosing foster care can be an emotionally challenging but compassionate decision, offering both time and support for mothers navigating complex circumstances.

What is Foster Care?

1. **Definition and Purpose**

   - **Foster care is a temporary living arrangement for children whose parents or guardians are unable to care for them due to personal, financial, or situational challenges.**

   - **It allows children to live in a safe and nurturing environment while parents receive the time or resources needed to make long-term decisions about their child's care.**

2. **Who Provides Foster Care?**

   - **Licensed Foster Families: Families who have undergone training and background checks to provide a stable and loving home for children.**

- o **Group Homes or Institutions: For older children or those with special needs, group homes staffed by professionals may serve as temporary housing.**

3. Why Choose Foster Care?

- o **Temporary Solution: Provides mothers with time to address financial, emotional, or personal challenges.**

- o **Safe Environment for the Child: Ensures the child is cared for while long-term plans are made.**

- o **Flexibility: Offers options for reunification, guardianship, or adoption based on the mother's decision and circumstances.**

The Process of Placing a Child in Foster Care

1. Contacting Child Welfare Services

- o **Begin by reaching out to your local Department of Child and Family Services (DCFS) or equivalent agency. They will guide you through the process and provide an overview of foster care options.**

2. Understanding Your Rights

- o **Voluntary Placement: In some cases, foster care can be arranged voluntarily, where you retain parental rights and work with social services to determine the best plan for your child.**

- o **Involuntary Placement: If foster care is court-ordered due to concerns for the child's safety, the process will** involve legal proceedings and case plans for reunification or alternative arrangements.

3. Developing a Care Plan

- Collaboration with Caseworkers: Social workers will work with you to create a care plan outlining the child's needs, visitation schedules, and steps toward reunification if desired.

- Reassessment of Circumstances: Regular reviews will assess whether reunification is possible or if other options like guardianship or adoption should be pursued.

4. Maintaining Contact with Your Child

- Depending on the situation, mothers may be allowed supervised or unsupervised visitation.

- Communication options, such as phone calls or letters, can help maintain a bond during the foster care period.

5. Transitioning to Long-Term Solutions

- Foster care allows mothers to decide whether they want to work toward reunification, explore guardianship, or consider adoption as a permanent solution for their child's future.

1. Emotional and Counseling Services

- Counseling Support: Placing a child in foster care can evoke feelings of guilt, loss, or uncertainty. Professional counseling can provide coping strategies and emotional healing.

- Peer Support Groups: Join groups where other mothers share their experiences with foster care. Knowing you are not alone can be a source of strength.

2. Caseworker Guidance

- Social workers play a vital role in helping mothers navigate the foster care system. They can provide:
  - Clear explanations of the process.
  - Assistance with legal and administrative requirements.
  - Emotional support and resources for the mother's well-being.

3. Legal Support

- Retain legal counsel or seek free legal aid services to understand your rights and options throughout the foster care process.

4. Community Resources

- Parenting Classes: Many communities offer programs to help mothers prepare for reunification or alternative parenting roles.

- o Housing and Financial Assistance: Programs like TANF or Section 8 can provide temporary support while you work toward stability.

5. **Faith-Based and Nonprofit Organizations**

- o **Many religious or nonprofit organizations provide foster care support services, including counseling, childcare assistance, and transitional housing for mothers.**

Choosing foster care is a compassionate decision that prioritizes the child's well-being while giving the mother space to address her circumstances. It provides time, structure, and support to explore long-term plans without immediate pressure.

While foster care may not be the right solution for everyone, it can be a vital resource for mothers seeking temporary support while navigating a difficult situation. By understanding the process, maintaining a connection with your child, and accessing available support networks, you can make choices that reflect care, courage, and love.

Foster care is not the end of a journey but a step toward clarity, healing, and a brighter future for both mother and child.

6. Turning to Family and Friends

In times of uncertainty, family and friends can serve as a vital support system, offering encouragement, practical assistance, and emotional strength. However, sharing your decision to continue a pregnancy and asking for help can feel overwhelming, especially when reactions may vary. This chapter provides strategies for effectively communicating your decision, navigating both supportive and unsupportive responses, and building a network of understanding and encouragement.

How to Share Your Decision and Ask for Help

1. **Prepare Yourself Before the Conversation**

   - **Take time to process your emotions and clarify your decision. Reflect on why you've chosen this path, and be confident in your reasoning.**

   - **Anticipate questions or concerns and prepare responses that communicate your needs and intentions clearly.**

2. **Choose the Right Time and Setting**

   - **Select a private and comfortable environment for these discussions, minimizing distractions and ensuring everyone involved feels at ease.**

- Timing matters; choose a moment when your loved ones are more likely to be receptive and available to talk.

3. **Be Honest and Direct**

   - Share your decision with openness and authenticity. Let them know how you arrived at your choice and what it means to you.

   - For example: *"I've decided to continue this pregnancy because it aligns with my values and hopes for the future. I want to share this with you because your support means so much to me."*

4. **Communicate Your Needs Clearly**

   - Explain how they can support you—whether it's emotional encouragement, practical assistance, or simply listening without judgment.

   - Be specific about the kind of help you need, such as attending prenatal appointments, helping with childcare planning, or offering a listening ear.

5. **Acknowledge Their Feelings**

   - Recognize that this news may bring up emotions for them as well. Acknowledging their feelings, even if they differ from yours, can foster mutual respect.

   - For example: *"I understand this might be unexpected for you, and it's okay to have mixed feelings. I just ask for your support as I move forward."*

1. When Reactions Are Supportive

- **Express Gratitude: Let supportive loved ones know how much their encouragement means to you. A simple thank-you can strengthen your connection and make them feel appreciated.**

- **Involve Them in the Journey: Invite supportive family members or friends to join you in milestones like ultrasounds, parenting classes, or planning for the future.**

- **Lean on Their Strength: Use their encouragement as a source of confidence, especially during challenging moments.**

2. When Reactions Are Unsupportive

- **Stay Grounded in Your Decision: Remember that this is your life and your choice. Negative reactions often stem from fear, misunderstanding, or personal biases, not from a lack of love.**

- **Set Boundaries: Politely but firmly establish boundaries if someone's negativity becomes overwhelming. For example: *"I respect your opinion, but I need support right now, not criticism."***

- Avoid Arguments: Instead of engaging in heated debates, focus on calmly reiterating your decision and redirecting the conversation if needed.

3. Balancing Mixed Reactions

- Acknowledge Concerns: If loved ones express doubt or worry, listen to their concerns without defensiveness. Respond with clarity and reassurance, helping them see your perspective.

- Look for Common Ground: Focus on shared values, such as wanting what's best for the baby or your future, to foster understanding and collaboration.

4. Seeking Outside Support When Needed

- If family or friends remain unsupportive, consider turning to external resources such as counselors, support groups, or community organizations. These networks can provide the understanding and encouragement you may not receive elsewhere.

Practical Tips for Strengthening Your Support Network

1. Create a Circle of Trusted Allies

- Identify family members or friends who consistently show understanding and compassion. Build your core support network around them.

- Recognize that not everyone needs to be involved. Prioritize quality over quantity in your relationships.

2. **Regularly Communicate Your Needs**

   - ○ **Keep your support network updated about your progress and needs. Open, ongoing communication fosters stronger bonds and ensures you receive timely assistance.**

3. **Offer Opportunities to Help**

   - ○ **Giving loved ones specific ways to support you—such as running errands, attending appointments, or simply checking in—can make them feel involved and valued.**

4. **Practice Self-Care in Relationships**

   - ○ **Protect your emotional well-being by setting boundaries with unsupportive individuals and focusing your energy on positive, uplifting connections.**

Final Thoughts on Turning to Family and Friends

Reaching out to loved ones during this time can provide invaluable emotional and practical support. While not every reaction may be positive, approaching conversations with confidence, clarity, and compassion can help build a foundation of understanding and collaboration.

Remember, your decision is a reflection of your strength and values. Surrounding yourself with those who respect and support your journey will empower you to move forward with resilience, hope, and love.

7. Counseling and Emotional Support

Navigating an unplanned pregnancy can bring a whirlwind of emotions—fear, confusion, anxiety, and sometimes isolation. Seeking counseling and emotional support is a powerful step toward finding clarity, healing, and resilience. Whether through professional services, support groups, or peer networks, these resources can help you process your emotions, build strength, and connect with others who understand your journey.

Finding Professional Counseling Services

1. The Benefits of Counseling

- Professional counselors provide a safe, judgment-free space to explore your thoughts and feelings.
- They can help you develop coping strategies, process complex emotions, and make informed decisions about your future.

2. Where to Find Counseling Services

- Pregnancy Resource Centers: Many centers offer free or low-cost counseling tailored to women experiencing unplanned pregnancies.
- Licensed Therapists: Look for mental health professionals specializing in women's health, pregnancy, or life transitions. Platforms like Psychology Today, BetterHelp, or Talkspace can help you find therapists in your area or online.

- Faith-Based Counseling: Religious organizations often provide counseling services that align with specific spiritual or moral values.

- Community Programs: Nonprofit organizations and local health departments frequently provide counseling services for low or no cost.

3. What to Expect in Counseling

- Exploring Your Emotions: A counselor will help you identify and validate your feelings, whether they're positive, negative, or somewhere in between.

- Setting Goals: Together, you'll work on setting emotional, practical, and personal goals to help you move forward.

- Learning Coping Skills: Techniques like mindfulness, journaling, or cognitive restructuring can help you manage stress and anxiety.

4. Tips for Choosing the Right Counselor

- Look for a professional who specializes in pregnancy-related concerns and aligns with your values.

- Don't be afraid to ask questions about their approach, experience, and availability during an initial consultation.

1. The Power of Community Support

- Support groups offer a space to connect with women facing similar situations. Sharing experiences fosters understanding, encouragement, and a sense of belonging.

- Group members often provide practical advice, emotional support, and firsthand insights into navigating pregnancy and its challenges.

2. Types of Support Groups

- In-Person Groups: Many community centers, hospitals, and pregnancy resource organizations host regular meetings for pregnant women.

- Online Communities: Virtual groups on platforms like Facebook, BabyCenter, or What to Expect provide 24/7 access to discussions, resources, and peer support.

- Specialized Groups: Some groups focus on specific needs, such as single mothers, women choosing adoption, or those experiencing financial hardship.

3. How to Find a Group

- Check with local pregnancy centers, churches, or healthcare providers for recommendations.

- o Search online for forums or social media groups tailored to pregnant women.

- o Ask other mothers or friends about groups they've found helpful.

4. Benefits of Joining

- o Gain practical advice from women who've walked a similar path.

- o Find emotional validation and encouragement during tough times.

- o Build lasting friendships with people who understand your journey.

The Role of Peer Networks in Providing Emotional Strength

1. What Are Peer Networks?

- o Peer networks are informal connections with people who've experienced or are experiencing similar challenges. These networks offer mutual support, empathy, and shared understanding.

2. Examples of Peer Networks

- o Motherhood Mentorships: Programs pairing expectant mothers with experienced moms for guidance and companionship.

- o Online Forums and Social Media: Virtual spaces where women share advice, encouragement, and real-life stories.

  - o Faith-Based Peer Groups: Church or temple groups that create a nurturing environment for pregnant women.

3. How Peer Networks Build Strength

  - o Shared Stories: Hearing others' journeys helps you realize you're not alone and provides perspective on your own situation.

  - o Practical Tips: From managing morning sickness to preparing for delivery, peers can share tried-and-true advice.

  - o Emotional Validation: Peers offer empathy and understanding that can't always be found elsewhere.

4. Building Your Own Peer Network

  - o Reach out to friends, family, or coworkers who've experienced pregnancy or parenthood.

  - o Join community events, prenatal classes, or local meetups to form connections.

  - o Stay open to building relationships with people from diverse backgrounds and experiences.

Counseling and peer support are invaluable tools for navigating the emotional complexities of pregnancy. Whether you choose to speak with a professional, join a support group, or connect informally with peers, these resources remind you that you don't have to face this journey alone.

Embracing the power of shared experiences and professional guidance can help you find clarity, strength, and hope. You deserve support, understanding, and compassion as you navigate this significant chapter of your life. By reaching out and building your network, you'll not only strengthen yourself but also find comfort in the collective wisdom and care of others.

8. Community Resources for Women

When facing an unplanned pregnancy, access to supportive community resources can make a significant difference. These organizations provide essential services, from medical care and counseling to housing and nourishment, ensuring that women receive the help they need to navigate their circumstances. Understanding and utilizing these resources can empower you to move forward with confidence and stability.

1. What Are Pregnancy Resource Centers?

- Pregnancy resource centers (PRCs) are nonprofit organizations dedicated to helping women facing unplanned pregnancies. They offer a wide range of free or low-cost services designed to provide emotional, medical, and practical support.

2. Services Offered by PRCs

- Pregnancy Testing and Ultrasounds: Many centers provide free pregnancy tests and ultrasounds to confirm the pregnancy and check on fetal development.

- Counseling and Emotional Support: PRCs often offer confidential counseling to help women explore their options and manage the emotional challenges of pregnancy.

- Parenting Classes: Learn essential parenting skills, from baby care to managing relationships and finances.

- Material Assistance: Some centers provide free items such as baby clothes, diapers, formula, and car seats to help with the immediate needs of new mothers.

- Adoption Referrals: PRCs can connect women with adoption agencies and offer guidance throughout the adoption process.

- Community Referrals: Many centers act as a bridge, connecting women to other local resources such as housing programs or healthcare providers.

3. **How to Find a Pregnancy Resource Center**

- Search online for PRCs in your area using directories like OptionLine.org or Care-Net.org.

- Ask healthcare providers or local churches for recommendations.

- Call national hotlines for assistance locating a nearby center.

Shelters, Food Banks, and Local Organizations

1. **Shelters and Transitional Housing**

- For women who need a safe place to stay, shelters and transitional housing programs offer short-term or long-term accommodations.

- Types of Shelters:
    - Women's shelters provide a secure environment for expectant mothers or those with children.

- Maternity homes focus specifically on pregnant women, offering housing, medical care, and life skills training.

- How to Access Shelter Services:

    - Contact local social services or dial 2-1-1 to find emergency housing options.

    - Reach out to organizations like Catholic Charities or Salvation Army, which often run shelters for women and families.

    - Ask pregnancy resource centers for referrals to maternity homes in your area.

2. Food Banks and Meal Programs

- Food banks and community kitchens ensure that women and families have access to nutritious meals, free of charge.

- How to Find Food Assistance:

    - Visit FeedingAmerica.org to locate nearby food banks.

    - Check local churches, community centers, or government websites for meal programs.

- Additional Resources:

    - Supplemental Nutrition Assistance Program (SNAP): Provides financial assistance for groceries.

- Women, Infants, and Children (WIC): Offers vouchers for nutritious foods and support for pregnant women and children under five.

3. **Local Organizations Offering Comprehensive Support**

   - Many local nonprofits provide a combination of services, including housing, medical care, and education.

   - Examples of Comprehensive Support Programs:

     - YWCA: Offers housing, counseling, and support for women and children.

     - United Way: Connects individuals to a broad range of community resources, including childcare and financial assistance.

     - Neighborhood Ministries: Community-based organizations often provide access to healthcare, legal aid, and mentorship programs.

Maximizing the Benefits of Community Resources

1. **Create a Resource Map**

   - Take note of the organizations in your area that offer assistance, and make a list of their services, locations, and contact information.

2. **Ask for Referrals**

- Many organizations work together to create a network of support. Don't hesitate to ask one organization to connect you with others that may be helpful.

3. **Be Prepared**

- When reaching out to community resources, have basic information on hand, such as your identification and details about your situation, to streamline the process.

4. **Follow Up**

- After receiving assistance, maintain communication with organizations that have been helpful. Building relationships can lead to continued support and resources in the future.

Final Thoughts on Community Resources for Women

Community resources are designed to offer a lifeline to women in need, providing not only material assistance but also emotional and practical support. By connecting with pregnancy resource centers, shelters, food banks, and local organizations, you can access the help necessary to navigate your current situation with greater ease and stability.

Remember, asking for help is a sign of strength, not weakness. These resources exist because you are not alone—there are people and organizations ready to stand by you and support your journey. By reaching out, you are taking a proactive step toward creating a brighter future for yourself and your child.

9. Financial Planning and Support

Raising a child involves significant financial responsibilities, but careful planning and access to available resources can make the journey manageable. Whether you're budgeting for the essentials, exploring government assistance programs, or finding affordable childcare options, this chapter provides practical tips and resources to help you plan effectively and confidently.

Budgeting for a Baby: Essentials and Tips

1. **Understanding Baby Essentials**

   - **Immediate Needs: Diapers, wipes, baby clothes, a crib or bassinet, and a car seat are some of the most crucial items for newborns.**

   - **Ongoing Expenses: Formula or breastfeeding supplies, baby food, healthcare, and childcare will be recurring costs.**

   - **Miscellaneous Items: Baby monitors, strollers, and toys are useful but can often be purchased second-hand or received as gifts.**

2. **Creating a Budget**

- o **Start with Essentials:** Make a list of the items you'll
     need before the baby arrives and their estimated
     costs.

- o **Separate One-Time and Recurring Costs:** This helps
     you plan for upfront expenses like a crib while
     preparing for ongoing needs like diapers.

- o **Track Income and Expenses:** Use budgeting apps or a
     simple spreadsheet to monitor your spending and
     identify areas where you can save.

3. Tips for Saving Money

- o **Borrow or Buy Second-Hand:** Many baby items, such
     as clothes and strollers, can be borrowed from friends
     or purchased gently used.

- o **Create a Baby Registry:** Let loved ones contribute by
     gifting essential items.

- o **Shop Sales and Use Coupons:** Look for discounts,
     especially on bulk purchases of diapers and wipes.

4. Planning for Unexpected Costs

- o **Emergency Fund:** Set aside a small amount each
     month for unexpected expenses, such as medical bills
     or extra childcare needs.

- o **Healthcare Costs:** Research your health insurance
     coverage to understand what prenatal and postnatal
     care is covered and budget for out-of-pocket
     expenses.

1. Women, Infants, and Children (WIC)

- **Overview: WIC provides nutritional support for pregnant women, breastfeeding mothers, and children under five.**

- **Benefits: Includes free or discounted access to healthy foods, nutrition education, and breastfeeding support.**

- **How to Apply: Visit your state's WIC website or a local health department to check eligibility and apply.**

2. Temporary Assistance for Needy Families (TANF)

- **Overview: TANF offers financial aid to low-income families, helping with necessities like food, housing, and childcare.**

- **Benefits: Cash assistance, job training, and support services to help families achieve financial independence.**

- **How to Apply: Contact your local Department of Human Services (DHS) or apply online through your state's TANF program.**

3. Medicaid and CHIP (Children's Health Insurance Program)

- **Overview: Medicaid provides free or low-cost healthcare for low-income pregnant women and their children. CHIP extends coverage to families with slightly higher incomes.

- o Benefits: Covers prenatal care, delivery, pediatric visits, vaccinations, and more.
- o How to Apply: Apply through your state's Medicaid office or healthcare marketplace.

4. Supplemental Nutrition Assistance Program (SNAP)

- o Overview: SNAP provides financial assistance for groceries to low-income families.
- o How to Apply: Visit your state's SNAP website or contact your local Department of Social Services.

Childcare Options and Subsidies

1. Affordable Childcare Options

- o Relatives or Friends: Trusted family members or friends can often provide affordable or free childcare.
- o Community Childcare Programs: Many local organizations offer reduced-cost daycare services for low-income families.
- o At-Home Daycare Providers: Licensed home-based providers are often less expensive than larger daycare centers.

2. Government Childcare Subsidies

- **Child Care and Development Fund (CCDF): A federal program providing financial assistance to low-income families for childcare.**
  - **How to Apply: Contact your state's childcare subsidy office for details and eligibility requirements.**
- **Head Start and Early Head Start: These programs offer free early childhood education, health, and nutrition services to eligible families.**
  - **How to Apply: Visit the Head Start website or contact a local program.**

3. **Tax Credits for Childcare**

- **Child Tax Credit: Provides financial relief for families with dependent children.**
- **Child and Dependent Care Credit: Offers tax savings for families paying for childcare services while working or attending school.**

4. **Tips for Managing Childcare Costs**

- **Look for Sliding Scale Fees: Many childcare providers adjust fees based on income.**
- **Share Childcare: Coordinate with other families to share babysitters or childcare costs.**
- **Employer Benefits: Check if your workplace offers childcare discounts or flexible spending accounts (FSAs) for childcare expenses.**

Planning for the financial aspects of raising a child can feel daunting, but with careful budgeting, assistance programs, and affordable childcare options, it is manageable. Remember, you don't have to face these challenges alone—many resources are available to help you provide for your child while maintaining financial stability.

By taking proactive steps and reaching out for support, you can create a secure and nurturing environment for your child, giving both of you the opportunity to thrive. The journey may require effort, but with determination and the right tools, you can confidently build a future filled with hope and possibility.

10. Healthcare During Pregnancy

Proper healthcare during pregnancy is vital for ensuring the health and well-being of both mother and baby. From accessing prenatal care to addressing maternal health needs and planning for postnatal recovery, understanding available resources and taking proactive steps can make a significant difference in your pregnancy journey.

1. What is Prenatal Care?

- Prenatal care involves regular medical check-ups, tests, and guidance to monitor the health of both the mother and the developing baby. It is critical for detecting and addressing potential complications early.

2. Where to Access Prenatal Care

- **Hospitals and Clinics:**
  - Most hospitals and community health clinics provide prenatal care, including routine exams, ultrasounds, and screenings.
- **OB-GYN or Midwife Services:**
  - Obstetricians specialize in pregnancy care and delivery, while midwives often provide a more personalized and holistic approach.
- **Federally Qualified Health Centers (FQHCs):**
  - These centers offer affordable or free prenatal care for low-income individuals, regardless of insurance status.
- **Low-Cost Options:**

- Planned Parenthood and local health departments often provide affordable prenatal care, especially for uninsured women.

3. **How to Get Started**

   - Schedule your first prenatal appointment as soon as you know you're pregnant.

   - Bring medical records and a list of any pre-existing conditions or medications.

   - Ask about costs upfront and explore payment options if uninsured.

4. **Financial Support for Prenatal Care**

   - Medicaid: Covers prenatal and maternity care for eligible low-income women.

   - Charitable Organizations: Groups like March of Dimes offer financial assistance for prenatal care.

   - Sliding Scale Clinics: Many clinics adjust fees based on income.

---

1. **Physical Health During Pregnancy**

   - Nutrition:

     - Eat a balanced diet rich in fruits, vegetables, lean proteins, and whole grains. Include prenatal vitamins with folic acid to support fetal development.

- o **Exercise:**
    - **Regular, moderate exercise, like walking or prenatal yoga, helps maintain physical health, reduce stress, and prepare for childbirth.**
    - **Consult your healthcare provider about safe activities for your pregnancy stage.**
- o **Sleep and Rest:**
    - **Prioritize rest and sleep to help your body recover and adapt to the physical demands of pregnancy.**
- o **Avoid Harmful Substances:**
    - **Avoid alcohol, tobacco, and recreational drugs, as they can harm your baby. If you need help quitting, seek support from your healthcare provider.**

2. Emotional Health During Pregnancy

- o **Managing Stress:**
    - **Practice mindfulness techniques like meditation, deep breathing, or journaling to reduce stress and anxiety.**
- o **Seek Emotional Support:**

- Share your feelings with trusted family, friends, or a counselor to process emotions and address any concerns.

  o **Monitor Mental Health:**

  - Be aware of mood changes that may indicate prenatal depression or anxiety. Speak to a healthcare provider if you experience persistent sadness, worry, or hopelessness.

3. **Key Screenings and Tests**

  o **Ultrasounds: Monitor the baby's growth and development.**

  o **Blood Tests: Detect conditions like anemia, gestational diabetes, and infections.**

  o **Genetic Testing: Available for mothers concerned about hereditary conditions.**

Postnatal Care for Mother and Baby

1. **What is Postnatal Care?**

  o **Postnatal care focuses on the health and recovery of the mother and the well-being of the newborn during the first six weeks after delivery.**

2. **Care for the Mother**

  o **Physical Recovery:**

- Healing from childbirth requires rest, hydration, and proper nutrition. For cesarean deliveries, follow specific recovery instructions provided by your doctor.
  - **Breastfeeding Support:**
    - Lactation consultants can provide guidance for successful breastfeeding. Many hospitals and clinics offer these services.
  - **Follow-Up Appointments:**
    - Schedule a postnatal check-up 4–6 weeks after delivery to assess physical and emotional recovery.
  - **Addressing Postpartum Depression:**
    - Seek help if you experience feelings of sadness, irritability, or emotional numbness, as these may indicate postpartum depression.

3. Care for the Baby

- **Newborn Check-Ups:**
  - The baby's first doctor's visit should occur within the first week of birth. Pediatricians will monitor weight gain, feeding, and overall health.
- **Immunizations:**

- Follow your healthcare provider's schedule for vaccines to protect your baby from preventable illnesses.
  - **Breastfeeding or Formula Feeding:**
    - Choose a feeding method that works best for you and your baby, ensuring they receive proper nutrition.

4. **Resources for Postnatal Care**

- **Home Visiting Programs: Many states offer home visits by nurses or counselors to assist with newborn care and maternal health.**
- **Support Groups: Connect with other new mothers for advice, encouragement, and companionship.**
- **Hotlines and Helplines: Organizations like Postpartum Support International provide resources and support for mental health concerns.**

Final Thoughts on Healthcare During Pregnancy

Taking care of your health and well-being during and after pregnancy is essential for both you and your baby. From accessing prenatal care to focusing on your physical and emotional needs, each step you take brings you closer to a healthy and fulfilling journey into motherhood.

Remember, there are many resources available to support you through every stage of this process. By seeking medical care,

prioritizing self-care, and reaching out for help when needed, you're ensuring the best possible start for you and your child.

11. Understanding Your Legal Rights

- Navigating the legal aspects of parenting can feel complex, but understanding your rights and responsibilities empowers you to make informed decisions. From custody arrangements to financial obligations and access to legal assistance, this chapter outlines the key legal considerations for parents and provides resources to guide you through the process.

11.   Custody and Parental Responsibilities

Types of Custody

- **Physical Custody: Refers to where the child lives and who is responsible for day-to-day care. It can be sole (one parent) or joint (shared between both parents).**

- **Legal Custody: Involves the right to make important decisions about the child's upbringing, such as education, healthcare, and religion. Like physical custody, this can also be sole or joint.**

Establishing Custody

- **For unmarried parents, custody is typically established through a legal process. In most states, mothers are presumed to have custody at birth unless a court orders otherwise.**

- **Fathers may need to establish paternity to gain custody or visitation rights, which can be done through voluntary acknowledgment or court-ordered genetic testing.**

Visitation Rights

- **Non-custodial parents often have visitation rights, which can be agreed upon mutually or outlined by a court order.**

- **Visitation schedules vary and can include supervised visits if there are safety concerns.**

Responsibilities of Custody

- **Custodial parents are responsible for providing a safe, nurturing environment for the child.**

- **Joint custody requires cooperation and communication between parents to make decisions in the child's best interest.**

Child Support and Financial Obligations

What is Child Support?

- **Child support is a financial contribution made by one parent to assist the other in covering the costs of raising a child. It is typically ordered when one parent has primary custody, and the other has visitation rights or limited custody.**

Calculating Child Support

Child support amounts are determined based on state guidelines, which consider factors such as:

Both parents' income

The child's needs (e.g., education, healthcare)

Custody arrangements and time spent with each parent

Many states use online calculators to estimate child support obligations.

Enforcing Child Support

If a parent fails to pay court-ordered child support, enforcement measures may include wage garnishment, tax refund interception, or license suspension.

It is important to keep records of payments and agreements to address disputes if they arise.

Financial Obligations Beyond Child Support

Non-custodial parents may also share responsibility for additional costs, such as:

Uninsured medical expenses

Extracurricular activities

College tuition (if agreed upon or ordered by the court)

Resources for Legal Assistance

Legal Aid Organizations

Many nonprofit organizations provide free or low-cost legal services to individuals with limited income.

Examples include:

Legal Aid Society: Offers assistance with family law issues, including custody and child support.

LawHelp.org: Connects individuals to local legal aid resources.

Family Law Attorneys

Hiring a family law attorney can provide personalized guidance on custody, child support, and other legal matters.

Some attorneys offer free consultations or work on a sliding scale based on income.

Court Resources

Most family courts provide self-help centers with resources for filing custody or child support cases.

Many courts also offer mediation services to help parents reach agreements without lengthy litigation.

Online Legal Assistance

Platforms like Rocket Lawyer and LegalZoom provide affordable legal documents and consultations.

State websites often offer free forms and instructions for filing family law cases.

Government Support Services

Child support enforcement agencies in each state help establish and enforce child support orders.

State departments of health or family services can assist with paternity establishment and custody agreements.

Tips for Navigating Legal Processes

Keep Detailed Records

Maintain documentation of custody arrangements, financial contributions, and any communication with the other parent.

These records can be crucial in court proceedings or disputes.

Communicate Clearly and Respectfully

When dealing with custody or child support matters, clear and respectful communication with the other parent can prevent misunderstandings and reduce conflict.

Know Your State Laws

Family law varies by state, so it's important to familiarize yourself with the specific regulations in your area.

Visit your state's court or government websites for accurate and up-to-date information.

Seek Support When Needed

Don't hesitate to consult a legal professional or reach out to support organizations if you feel overwhelmed or unsure of your rights.

Final Thoughts on Understanding Your Legal Rights

- **Understanding your legal rights and responsibilities is a critical part of navigating parenthood. Whether you're establishing custody, ensuring financial stability through child support, or seeking legal assistance, being informed empowers you to make decisions that protect both you and your child.**

- **Remember, help is available through legal aid organizations, family courts, and community resources. With the right support and knowledge, you can navigate these processes confidently and create a secure foundation for your family's future.**

12. Coping with Stress and Anxiety

Pregnancy, especially when faced with challenging circumstances, can bring heightened feelings of stress and anxiety. Learning how to manage these emotions is vital for your overall well-being and the health of your baby. This chapter provides practical tools, from mindfulness practices and journaling prompts to self-care strategies, to help you find calm, clarity, and strength during this transformative time.

Mindfulness Practices and Breathing Exercises

1. **What is Mindfulness?**

   - **Mindfulness is the practice of being fully present in the moment without judgment. It helps you focus on the here and now rather than being overwhelmed by past worries or future uncertainties.**

2. **Simple Mindfulness Practices**

   - **Body Scan Meditation: Lie down or sit comfortably and slowly focus your attention on each part of your body, starting from your toes and moving upward. Acknowledge any tension and gently release it.**

   - **Mindful Walks: Spend time walking in nature, focusing on your senses—what you see, hear, smell, and feel. This helps ground you in the present moment.**

- Gratitude Practice: Each day, take a moment to list three things you're grateful for. This simple act can shift your focus from anxiety to positivity.

3. **Breathing Exercises to Reduce Anxiety**

   - **Deep Belly Breathing:** Place one hand on your belly and the other on your chest. Inhale deeply through your nose, allowing your belly to expand. Exhale slowly through your mouth. Repeat for several minutes.

   - **Box Breathing:** Inhale for a count of 4, hold your breath for 4, exhale for 4, and hold again for 4. Repeat this cycle to calm your nervous system.

   - **4-7-8 Breathing:** Inhale for a count of 4, hold for 7, and exhale slowly for 8. This technique promotes relaxation and reduces stress.

Journaling Prompts for Emotional Clarity

1. **The Benefits of Journaling**

   - **Writing down your thoughts and feelings can help you process emotions, gain perspective, and identify solutions to challenges.**

2. **Journaling Prompts**

   - *What emotions am I experiencing today, and why might I be feeling this way?*

   - *What are three things I can do to bring myself comfort or joy right now?*

- o *What am I most worried about, and what steps can I take to address these concerns?*

  - o *What positive qualities do I see in myself that will help me navigate this journey?*

  - o *What does my ideal future look like, and how can I take small steps toward it?*

3. **Tips for Effective Journaling**

   - o **Write Freely:** Don't worry about grammar or structure—just let your thoughts flow.

   - o **Be Honest:** Use your journal as a safe space to express emotions without fear of judgment.

   - o **Revisit Entries:** Reflecting on past entries can reveal growth and recurring themes, helping you understand yourself better.

4. **Creative Journaling**

   - o **If writing feels overwhelming, try alternative methods like sketching, creating lists, or writing letters to your future self or baby.**

Self-Care Strategies for Mental Health

1. **Prioritize Rest and Relaxation**

   - o **Adequate Sleep: Aim for 7–9 hours of sleep per night to allow your body and mind to recharge.**

- Unplug: Take breaks from technology and social media to reduce overstimulation and focus on calming activities.
- Soothing Rituals: Create a nightly routine, such as a warm bath, reading, or listening to calming music, to signal to your body that it's time to relax.

2. Maintain a Healthy Lifestyle

- Nutritious Diet: Eat a balanced diet rich in whole foods, fruits, and vegetables to nourish both your body and mind.
- Gentle Exercise: Activities like yoga, walking, or swimming release endorphins, improving mood and reducing stress. Always consult your doctor before starting new exercises during pregnancy.

3. Connect with Others

- Talk to trusted friends or family members who can provide a listening ear and emotional support.
- Join local or online support groups to connect with women experiencing similar challenges. Shared experiences can foster understanding and encouragement.

4. Practice Self-Compassion

- Be kind to yourself. Acknowledge that it's okay to feel overwhelmed or unsure.
- Replace negative self-talk with affirmations like:

- *I am doing the best I can.*

- *I am capable and resilient.*

- *This is a challenging time, but I will get through it.*

5. **Engage in Joyful Activities**

   o Set aside time for hobbies or activities that bring you joy, whether it's painting, cooking, reading, or spending time in nature.

6. **Seek Professional Support**

   o If stress or anxiety feels unmanageable, consider reaching out to a counselor or therapist. They can provide tools and techniques to help you navigate your emotions more effectively.

Final Thoughts on Coping with Stress and Anxiety

Coping with stress and anxiety during pregnancy requires a combination of self-awareness, supportive practices, and intentional care. Mindfulness, journaling, and self-care are powerful tools to help you regain a sense of calm and control.

Remember, you don't have to face this journey alone. Lean on trusted loved ones, seek support when needed, and be gentle with yourself as you navigate this transformative time. Each step you take toward managing stress is a step toward a healthier, more peaceful future for you and your baby.

13. Affirmations and Positive Thinking

Affirmations and positive thinking are powerful tools that can help shift your mindset, reduce stress, and build resilience. By cultivating a supportive inner dialogue, you can transform negative self-talk into empowering beliefs and strengthen your ability to face challenges. This chapter explores the importance of affirmations, how to create them, and provides examples to inspire strength and positivity.

Cultivating a Supportive Inner Dialogue

1. The Power of Your Inner Voice

- ○ **Your inner dialogue shapes how you view yourself and the world around you. Positive self-talk can foster confidence and hope, while negative self-talk can fuel doubt and fear.**

- ○ **Becoming aware of your thoughts allows you to challenge and replace unhelpful patterns with empowering ones.**

2. Recognizing Negative Self-Talk

- ○ **Common forms of negative self-talk include:**

  - ▪ *Catastrophizing*: **"I can't handle this."**

  - ▪ *Self-Criticism*: **"I'm not good enough."**

  - ▪ *Overgeneralization*: **"Nothing ever works out for me."**

o   When you catch yourself thinking negatively, pause and question the validity of those thoughts.

3. Reframing Negative Thoughts

o   **Replace limiting beliefs with constructive ones. For example:**

- Instead of: *"I'm not strong enough to handle this,"* say: *"I am capable of facing challenges and growing stronger."*

- Instead of: *"I always fail,"* say: *"Every setback is a chance to learn and improve."*

4. Creating Space for Positivity

o   **Spend time each day focusing on what you're grateful for, celebrating small victories, and acknowledging your efforts.**

o   **Surround yourself with uplifting influences, such as inspiring books, music, or supportive people who encourage positive thinking.**

Examples of Affirmations for Strength and Resilience

1. General Affirmations for Positivity

o   *I am worthy of love, respect, and support.*

o   *I trust myself to make the best decisions for me and my child.*

o   *I am capable of creating a fulfilling and meaningful life.*

2. **Affirmations for Managing Stress and Anxiety**

   - *I release what I cannot control and focus on what I can.*

   - *With each breath, I feel calmer and more at peace.*

   - *I have the strength to overcome any challenge that comes my way.*

3. **Affirmations for Emotional Resilience**

   - *I am allowed to feel my emotions without judgment.*

   - *Every challenge I face makes me stronger and more resilient.*

   - *I can navigate this journey with courage and grace.*

4. **Affirmations for Pregnancy and Motherhood**

   - *My body is capable of nurturing and supporting life.*

   - *I am learning and growing as a mother every day.*

   - *I am connected to my child in a bond of love and strength.*

5. **Affirmations for Self-Worth**

   - *I am enough, just as I am.*

   - *I deserve kindness, compassion, and understanding—from myself and others.*

   - *My worth is not defined by my circumstances, but by who I am.*

6. **Affirmations for Building Confidence**

- ○ *I have the power to create the life I desire.*

- ○ *I am strong, capable, and resourceful.*

- ○ *I trust myself to handle whatever comes my way.*

---

1. **Repeat Them Daily**

   - ○ **Practice saying affirmations aloud, writing them in a journal, or posting them where you'll see them often (e.g., on a mirror or phone wallpaper).**

2. **Engage with Emotion**

   - ○ **When reciting affirmations, connect with their meaning. Feel the emotions of strength, love, or peace as if the affirmation is already true.**

3. **Customize Affirmations to Your Needs**

   - ○ **Tailor affirmations to address specific challenges or areas where you need encouragement.**

4. **Use Affirmations During Stressful Moments**

   - ○ **When you feel overwhelmed, pause and repeat a calming affirmation to refocus your mind. For example: *"I am safe. I am loved. I am in control of my breath and my thoughts."***

Final Thoughts on Affirmations and Positive Thinking

Your thoughts have the power to shape your reality. By cultivating a supportive inner dialogue and embracing affirmations, you can create a mental environment of strength, resilience, and hope.

Remember, positive thinking doesn't mean ignoring challenges—it means choosing to believe in your ability to overcome them. Every time you replace self-doubt with self-belief, you take a step closer to becoming the best version of yourself. Start today with a single affirmation and watch how it transforms your mindset and your journey.

14. Personal Testimonials

Sharing real-life stories from women who have navigated challenging circumstances can provide inspiration, understanding, and hope. Whether through parenting, adoption, or finding support, these testimonials highlight the strength and resilience of women who have made life-affirming choices.

Stories from Women Who Chose Parenting

1. **Emily's Journey to Motherhood**
   "When I found out I was pregnant, I was terrified. I had no idea how I would manage financially or emotionally. But with the support of my family and a local pregnancy resource center, I found my footing. I learned how to budget, took parenting classes, and received emotional counseling. Today, I can't imagine my life without my son. He's my greatest joy and my reason to keep striving."

2. **Sophia's Story of Growth**
   "Being a single mom was never in my plans, but I made the choice to parent. It hasn't been easy, but every challenge has taught me something new about myself. I've learned to be resourceful, patient, and strong. The love I have for my daughter makes every sacrifice worthwhile."

---

1. **Sarah's Open Adoption Experience**
   "Choosing adoption was the hardest decision of my life, but I knew it was the right one for my baby and me. I chose an open adoption, which allows me to stay connected. I receive photos and updates, and I know my child is thriving with a loving family. While I still have moments of sadness, I feel peace knowing I gave him the best start possible."

2. **Maria's Story of Healing**
   "I wasn't ready to be a mom, but I wanted my baby to have every opportunity. I worked with a supportive adoption agency that helped me find a family who shared my values. Letting go was painful, but it was also healing. I know I made a choice out of love, and that brings me comfort."

Stories of Resilience from Women Who Found Support

1. **Jessica's Support Network**
   "I felt so alone when I found out I was pregnant. I didn't think I could do it. Then I found a support group for expectant mothers, and it changed everything. The women I met became like sisters to me—we shared advice, tears, and encouragement. With their help, I felt empowered to face every obstacle."

2. **Tamara's Journey to Stability**
   "When I lost my job while pregnant, I was sure I'd hit rock bottom. But a local community center stepped in to help me find housing, get access to food assistance, and

prepare for my baby. Today, I'm working again and providing for my son. I'll always be grateful for the support I found during my hardest moments."

Final Thoughts on Personal Testimonials

These stories show that while every journey is unique, the common threads of love, resilience, and support run through them all. Whether choosing to parent, pursuing adoption, or seeking help, these women found strength in their decisions and in the resources available to them.

Their experiences remind us that, even in the face of uncertainty, hope and courage can lead to profound transformation. You are not alone—there is a network of support, and your journey can inspire others just as theirs have.

15. Recommended Reading and Media

Finding the right resources can provide invaluable insights, guidance, and encouragement during your journey. This section highlights recommended books, articles, and other media to support you in areas such as parenting, adoption, and emotional well-being. These resources are carefully selected to empower, inform, and inspire you as you navigate this transformative time.

Books on Parenting, Adoption, and Emotional Healing

1. **Parenting**

   - ***What to Expect When You're Expecting*** **by Heidi Murkoff**

     - **A comprehensive guide to pregnancy, addressing everything from prenatal care to preparing for delivery.**

   - ***Parenting with Love and Logic*** **by Charles Fay and Foster Cline**

     - **Offers strategies for raising responsible, well-adjusted children with compassion and consistency.**

   - ***The Whole-Brain Child*** **by Daniel J. Siegel and Tina Payne Bryson**

- Explains how to nurture your child's emotional and cognitive development using neuroscience-backed techniques.

2. Adoption

- *Adoption: Choosing It, Living It, Loving It* by Dr. Ray Guarendi
  - A practical and heartwarming guide for birth mothers and adoptive families.
- *The Open-Hearted Way to Open Adoption* by Lori Holden
  - Offers insights into navigating open adoption with transparency, respect, and love.
- *Adoption Is a Family Affair!* by Patricia Irwin Johnston
  - A guide for explaining adoption to family and friends, ensuring their support and understanding.

3. Emotional Healing

- *Self-Compassion: The Proven Power of Being Kind to Yourself* by Dr. Kristin Neff
  - A transformative book on embracing self-compassion to heal and grow through life's challenges.
- *Rising Strong* by Brené Brown

- A powerful exploration of resilience, focusing on how to recover and thrive after setbacks.

  - *Mindful Motherhood: Practical Tools for Staying Sane During Pregnancy and Your Child's First Year* by Cassandra Vieten

    - Combines mindfulness practices with practical advice to help manage the emotional ups and downs of motherhood.

Articles Offering Practical Advice and Emotional Support

1. **Parenting**

   - "10 Must-Know Tips for New Moms" (*Parents Magazine*)

     - Offers simple and effective advice for first-time mothers adjusting to life with a newborn.

   - "How to Build a Parenting Support Network" (*Today's Parent*)

     - Guides mothers on creating a strong network of emotional and practical support.

   - "The Importance of Bonding with Your Baby" (*Verywell Family*)

     - Explores ways to foster a strong emotional connection with your newborn.

2. **Adoption**

- o **"Understanding the Adoption Process: A Guide for Birth Mothers"** (*American Adoptions*)
  - **Breaks down the steps of adoption and offers insights into choosing the right path.**
- o **"Open vs. Closed Adoption: Pros and Cons"** (*Adoption.com*)
  - **Provides a balanced look at different types of adoption to help mothers make informed decisions.**
- o **"How to Handle the Emotional Side of Adoption"** (*PsychCentral*)
  - **Offers advice for coping with grief, acceptance, and finding peace after placing a child for adoption.**

3. Emotional Healing

- o **"How to Practice Self-Care During Pregnancy"** (*Healthline*)
  - **Practical tips for nurturing your emotional and physical well-being.**
- o **"Journaling for Stress Relief: How Writing Can Improve Your Mood"** (*Psychology Today*)
  - **Explains the benefits of journaling and offers prompts to help you get started.**

- o "Mindfulness Techniques to Reduce Stress and Anxiety" (*Mindful.org*)

  - Provides beginner-friendly exercises for staying grounded and present.

How to Use These Resources

1. **Choose Based on Your Needs**

   - o Whether you're seeking advice on parenting, exploring adoption, or working on emotional healing, select resources that address your immediate concerns and interests.

2. **Take Notes and Reflect**

   - o As you read or engage with these materials, jot down key takeaways and how they relate to your situation. Reflecting on these insights can help you internalize and apply them effectively.

3. **Share with Your Support Network**

   - o Share articles or books with family, friends, or a support group. Discussing these resources can deepen understanding and foster meaningful conversations.

4. **Access Online or In-Person**

   - o Many of these books are available through local libraries, bookstores, or online retailers. Articles can often be accessed for free on reputable websites.

Final Thoughts on Recommended Reading and Media

The journey of parenting, adoption, or personal growth can feel overwhelming, but you don't have to navigate it alone. These carefully chosen resources provide the guidance, knowledge, and inspiration you need to face challenges with confidence and clarity.

Remember, every step you take to learn, reflect, and grow brings you closer to a brighter future for yourself and your child. Let these resources be your companions, offering encouragement and wisdom as you move forward.

16. Essential Contacts

Having access to the right resources can be crucial when navigating the challenges of pregnancy, parenting, adoption, or emotional well-being. This section provides important contacts—hotlines for counseling, websites for local and national resources, and organizations offering free or low-cost services. These resources are designed to guide, support, and empower you during this transformative journey.

16. Hotlines for Counseling and Pregnancy Support

1. **National Pregnancy Helpline**

   - **Phone: 1-800-550-4900**
   - **Description: A 24/7 helpline offering pregnancy-related support, including counseling, adoption information, and referrals to local resources. The helpline is available in multiple languages.**

2. **Planned Parenthood Helpline**

   - **Phone: 1-800-230-7526**
   - **Description: Provides confidential information about pregnancy options, sexual health, and reproductive care. Offers referrals to local clinics for counseling and medical support.**

3. **Postpartum Support International**

   - **Phone: 1-800-944-4773**
   - **Description: A helpline for women experiencing postpartum depression or anxiety. Provides support, counseling, and resources for both new mothers and their families.**

4. **National Domestic Violence Hotline**

   - **Phone: 1-800-799-7233 (SAFE)**
   - **Description: Confidential support for individuals in abusive relationships. Offers assistance in creating**

safety plans, providing resources, and connecting individuals to shelters.

5. Text 4Baby

   - Text: "Baby" to 511411

   - Description: A free service offering pregnancy and parenting tips via text messages. Information includes health care reminders, tips on prenatal and postnatal care, and resources for expectant mothers.

Websites for Local and National Resources

1. **American Pregnancy Association**

   - **Website:** www.americanpregnancy.org

   - **Description: Offers a wide range of information on pregnancy, parenting, miscarriage, and adoption. The site also includes directories for finding pregnancy centers, counselors, and other essential services.**

2. **National Adoption Center**

   - **Website:** www.adopt.org

   - **Description: Provides resources for women considering adoption, including information on the adoption process, types of adoption, and connecting with agencies.**

3. **BabyCenter**

   - **Website:** www.babycenter.com

- o Description: A trusted resource for parenting and pregnancy, BabyCenter offers articles, tools, and community forums. It also provides expert advice, including emotional and practical tips for new parents.

4. **National Women's Law Center**

- o Website: www.nwlc.org

- o Description: Provides legal resources and advocacy for women's rights, including family leave, pregnancy discrimination, and reproductive health care.

5. **United Way 2-1-1**

- o Website: www.211.org

- o Description: A national database that connects individuals with local resources, including food assistance, housing support, health care, and childcare. You can also call 2-1-1 for referrals to community services.

6. **March of Dimes**

- o Website: www.marchofdimes.org

- o Description: Focuses on improving the health of mothers and babies through education and advocacy. The site offers resources on pregnancy care, preterm birth, and healthy pregnancies.

1. Local Pregnancy Resource Centers

- Description: Many local pregnancy centers offer free pregnancy tests, counseling, adoption referrals, and baby supplies such as diapers, clothing, and formula. These centers are often volunteer-run and provide services confidentially.

- How to Find: Search online or visit sites like OptionLine to locate pregnancy centers near you.

2. The Salvation Army

- Website: www.salvationarmyusa.org

- Description: Offers a variety of services for women, including emergency shelter, food assistance, counseling, and maternal health services. They also run thrift stores where baby supplies are often available at low cost.

3. Catholic Charities USA

- Website: www.catholiccharitiesusa.org

- Description: Provides services to low-income families, including housing, food, financial assistance, and emotional support. Their programs are available regardless of religious affiliation.

4. WIC (Women, Infants, and Children Program)

- Website: www.fns.usda.gov/wic

- Description: Offers nutritional assistance to low-income pregnant women, breastfeeding mothers, and children under five. WIC provides free nutritious foods, counseling, and referrals to healthcare services.

5. **National Diaper Bank Network**

    - **Website:** www.nationaldiaperbanknetwork.org

    - **Description:** Connects individuals with local diaper banks to provide free or low-cost diapers for families in need. Diaper banks are often located in community centers, churches, and health organizations.

6. **Help Me Grow**

    - **Website:** www.helpmegrow.org

    - **Description:** A national program that connects families to developmental screenings, services, and resources for children, including referrals to medical care, nutrition programs, and early childhood education.

Final Thoughts on Essential Contacts

Having the right resources at your fingertips is crucial for navigating any challenging situation. These hotlines, websites, and organizations offer support, guidance, and practical help, ensuring that you have access to the resources you need to care for yourself and your baby.

Remember, reaching out for help is a powerful step toward building a brighter future. Whether you need emotional support, financial assistance, or practical resources, there are compassionate people and organizations ready to stand by you. You don't have to go through this journey alone.

17. Setting Personal Goals

Setting personal goals is a powerful way to create a vision for your future and take active steps toward achieving it. Whether you're navigating pregnancy, parenting, or personal transformation, goal-setting helps you focus on what's important and maintain motivation during challenging times. This chapter provides strategies for envisioning life after pregnancy and offers tools to help you build a fulfilling future, no matter where you are on your journey.

Envisioning Life After Pregnancy

1. **Creating a Vision for Your Future**

   - **Take a moment to think about the life you want to create after your pregnancy. This is not just about the immediate future, but also about how you see yourself, your family, and your goals in the coming years.**

   - **Visualize your life with the baby—what are your dreams for your family? What kind of environment do you want to provide for your child? Think about your personal growth and the kind of person you want to become.**

2. **Identifying Your Core Values**

- What do you value most? Is it your career, personal well-being, relationships, creativity, or service to others? Identifying your core values will help you align your goals with what truly matters to you.

- Consider how your vision for life after pregnancy can reflect these values. For example, if family is a priority, you might set goals around spending quality time with your child or creating a stable and loving home.

3. Setting Short-Term and Long-Term Goals

- Short-Term Goals: These are goals you can achieve in the near future (within weeks or months) and will help you adjust to life post-pregnancy. Examples include establishing a routine, learning new parenting skills, or returning to work or school.

- Long-Term Goals: These goals are more aspirational and can take years to accomplish. They might include advancing in your career, furthering your education, or creating a sustainable lifestyle for you and your family.

4. Embracing Flexibility

- Life after pregnancy may not always unfold exactly as planned, and that's okay. Setbacks and unexpected changes are a part of the journey. Stay flexible and adjust your goals as needed. Your vision is a guide, not a rigid map.

1. Breaking Down Goals into Actionable Steps

- Once you have a vision for your future, break down larger goals into smaller, achievable tasks. This makes the process less overwhelming and more manageable.

- For example, if your long-term goal is to go back to school, your smaller steps might include researching programs, applying for financial aid, and setting aside time for studying.

2. Creating a Timeline

- Set realistic timelines for your goals. Think about when you want to accomplish certain milestones and create a schedule that works for you. This could be a monthly or yearly plan.

- Use a planner, calendar, or goal-setting app to track your progress and keep yourself accountable.

3. Building a Support System

- Surround yourself with people who encourage your personal growth and support your goals. This could be family, friends, mentors, or support groups.

- Having a support system keeps you motivated, helps you stay on track, and provides emotional encouragement when you face challenges.

4. Developing New Skills

- Life after pregnancy may require new skills—whether that's parenting, balancing work and home life, or learning about personal finance.

- Consider taking courses, attending workshops, or reading books on topics that interest you. Invest in yourself to build the skills needed for your future.

5. Prioritizing Self-Care and Well-Being

- Building a fulfilling future begins with taking care of your mental, emotional, and physical health. Make self-care a priority by incorporating healthy habits like exercise, nutritious eating, and quality rest into your daily routine.

- Regularly reflect on your emotional and mental well-being. Take time to recharge and engage in activities that bring you joy and relaxation.

6. Visualizing Success

- Visualization is a powerful tool that can help you stay motivated and focused on your goals. Take time each day to imagine yourself successfully reaching your goals, whether it's seeing yourself excel in your career or enjoying a peaceful, joyful life with your child.

- Use vision boards, vision journals, or guided meditations to help keep your aspirations in focus.

1. **Celebrate Small Wins**

   - Every step forward, no matter how small, is progress. Celebrate your achievements along the way. This reinforces your commitment and builds confidence.

2. **Adjust and Refine Your Goals**

   - As life changes, so too may your goals. Revisit your goals regularly and adjust them as needed to reflect new priorities or circumstances.

3. **Practice Gratitude**

   - Incorporate gratitude into your daily routine. Reflect on the positive aspects of your life and the progress you've made. Gratitude fosters positivity and strengthens your resolve.

4. **Be Kind to Yourself**

   - Pursuing big goals takes time and patience. Don't be discouraged by setbacks or mistakes. Treat yourself with the same kindness and encouragement you would offer a friend.

Final Thoughts on Setting Personal Goals

Setting personal goals gives you the direction and focus needed to create the future you envision. Life after pregnancy may be challenging, but by taking small, intentional steps toward your goals, you can build a fulfilling, empowered future for yourself and your child.

Remember, the path to achieving your dreams is rarely linear, but with clarity, resilience, and the right tools, you can create a future that aligns with your values, aspirations, and the love you have for your family. Embrace the journey, and know that each step you take is a meaningful one toward becoming the best version of yourself.

18. Empowerment and Resilience

Empowerment and resilience are key to navigating life's most difficult moments, and they are within your reach, no matter what challenges you face. This chapter explores powerful stories of women who thrived despite adversity and provides practical strategies for building confidence, resilience, and finding your inner strength.

---

1. **Maya's Story of Overcoming Adversity**
   "When I found out I was pregnant, I was living paycheck to paycheck and barely able to make ends meet. I thought about all the obstacles, but I decided I wasn't going to let fear define my future. I reached out for help, connected with a support group, and took small steps each day to improve my situation. It wasn't easy, but now I'm thriving— working a job I love and raising my son with confidence."

2. **Rebecca's Journey to Resilience**
   "I was a single mom when I found out I was pregnant with my second child. There were days when I didn't know how I was going to keep going, but I kept telling myself that I was strong enough. I found a local program for single mothers, where I learned budgeting, parenting skills, and received emotional support. Today, I'm not just surviving—I'm thriving, and I'm so proud of the family I've built."

3. **Alicia's Story of Rising Above**
   "Being a young mom without family support seemed impossible, but I never gave up. I worked hard, got my education, and took control of my future. Today, I'm an advocate for young mothers, helping them find their own paths to success. It's amazing to see how far I've come, and now I'm dedicated to helping others overcome their challenges."

---

1. Embrace Your Journey

- **Recognize Your Progress:** It's easy to focus on what's not going right, but take a moment each day to reflect on your progress. Small victories, like taking care of yourself, handling a difficult situation, or seeking help, show your resilience and growth.

- **Celebrate Your Strengths:** Identify your strengths, whether they're emotional resilience, problem-solving, or empathy, and recognize them in your daily life. Confidence comes from recognizing your own value.

2. Shift Your Perspective

- **Reframe Challenges:** Instead of seeing obstacles as roadblocks, view them as opportunities to learn, grow, and become more resilient. Challenges don't define you—they refine you.

- Self-Talk Matters: The way you speak to yourself can shape your experience. Replace negative thoughts like "I can't do this" with empowering affirmations like "I am capable," "I am resourceful," or "I will get through this."

3. **Build a Supportive Network**

   - Surround Yourself with Uplifting People: Your circle of support can make a huge difference in building confidence. Seek out people who encourage, motivate, and help you see your potential.

   - Connect with Like-minded Individuals: Join groups, support circles, or communities where you can share experiences, offer encouragement, and receive support. When you feel supported, it becomes easier to stay resilient.

4. **Practice Self-Compassion**

   - Be Gentle with Yourself: Life is filled with ups and downs. Treat yourself with the same kindness and understanding you would offer a close friend. Acknowledge that it's okay to have setbacks and that you are doing your best.

   - Recognize Your Efforts: Take time to acknowledge the hard work you're putting into managing your responsibilities. Recognizing your own effort builds inner strength and boosts self-confidence.

5. Set Boundaries and Prioritize Your Well-Being

- Learn to Say No: Setting healthy boundaries is a powerful way to protect your energy and maintain resilience. Don't be afraid to say no to things that drain you or take away from your personal well-being.

- Prioritize Self-Care: Whether it's through physical activity, relaxation, hobbies, or alone time, caring for yourself allows you to recharge and come back stronger. Your mental and emotional health is just as important as anything else in your life.

Resilience Strategies for Building a Fulfilling Life

1. Visualize Your Success

- Take a few moments every day to visualize yourself achieving your goals, overcoming challenges, and becoming the person you want to be. Visualizing success helps build the mental resilience necessary to stay motivated.

2. Practice Gratitude

- Start or end each day by writing down three things you're grateful for. Gratitude shifts your focus to what's going well, creating a positive mindset that strengthens resilience and fosters confidence.

3. **Focus on What You Can Control**

   - Life often brings unpredictability, but you have the power to control how you react to situations. Focusing on what you can control, like your mindset, actions, and reactions, strengthens your ability to face challenges with resilience.

4. **Seek Professional Help When Needed**

   - There is no shame in seeking help when you need it. A therapist, counselor, or coach can provide invaluable tools for managing stress, improving self-esteem, and building emotional resilience.

Final Thoughts on Empowerment and Resilience

Empowerment and resilience are cultivated over time through self-awareness, support, and taking proactive steps to build a strong foundation for your future. Every challenge is an opportunity for growth, and with each setback, you become stronger, more confident, and better equipped to handle whatever life brings.

Remember, your journey is uniquely yours. Embrace your strength, trust in your ability to navigate obstacles, and know that you have the power to create a fulfilling, empowered future. You are resilient, capable, and deserving of every success that lies ahead.

19. Parenting and Personal Development Classes

Investing in parenting and personal development classes can be an empowering way to prepare for the challenges of raising a child and building a fulfilling future. These workshops and programs provide valuable tools, knowledge, and skills that can enhance your parenting abilities, financial well-being, and overall personal growth. This chapter explores the importance of learning and growing as a parent and individual, and highlights key resources to support you on this journey.

Workshops on Parenting Skills and Emotional Intelligence

1. **Parenting Skills Workshops**

   - **Building Strong Foundations: Parenting workshops often focus on core skills such as discipline, effective communication, and understanding child development.**

   - **Positive Discipline: Learn non-punitive strategies to guide children's behavior and foster a positive parent-child relationship. Workshops often teach techniques that avoid yelling or punishment and instead emphasize connection and problem-solving.**

   - **Child Development Education: Gain insight into the developmental stages of your child's growth, from infancy through adolescence. Understanding** milestones can help you anticipate needs and challenges as your child matures.

2. Emotional Intelligence in Parenting

- What is Emotional Intelligence (EQ)?: Emotional intelligence involves the ability to identify, understand, and manage your emotions and the emotions of others. In parenting, EQ helps parents respond thoughtfully to their children's emotional needs, fostering empathy, self-regulation, and social skills.

- Workshops for Building EQ: Many parenting courses include components on developing emotional intelligence in both the parent and the child. These workshops teach how to model emotional awareness and coping strategies, helping your child grow emotionally healthy.

- Benefits of Emotional Intelligence: Parents who develop strong emotional intelligence are better equipped to handle stress, model emotional regulation, and build deeper connections with their children.

3. Where to Find Parenting Workshops

- Local Community Centers: Many cities offer parenting workshops through community centers, libraries, or churches. These can be a great place to find low-cost or free resources.

- o **Online Courses: Websites like Coursera, Udemy, and Khan Academy offer courses on parenting and child development, making it easy to learn at your own pace.**

- o **Nonprofit Organizations: Organizations like the Parenting Education Network or Parents as Teachers offer in-person or virtual classes that focus on parenting skills and family dynamics.**

---

1. Understanding Financial Literacy

- o **Why It Matters: Financial literacy is essential for managing your money, building savings, and planning for your child's future. Learning how to budget, save, and invest can reduce financial stress and help create a stable foundation for you and your family.**

- o **Basic Principles: Topics covered in financial literacy programs often include saving, budgeting, debt management, credit scores, and financial goal setting.**

2. Budgeting for Families

- o **Creating a Family Budget: Workshops often teach practical techniques for budgeting, such as the 50/30/20 rule (50% for needs, 30% for wants, and 20% for savings). Understanding how to allocate income properly can help families manage expenses and avoid financial stress.**

- Emergency Savings: Learn how to build an emergency fund to handle unexpected expenses, which is especially important when you have a child.

- Debt Management: Many programs focus on creating strategies to reduce debt, such as credit card payments or student loans, to ease financial burdens.

3. Where to Find Financial Literacy Classes

- Nonprofits and Community Organizations: Groups like Junior Achievement, The United Way, or local credit unions often offer free or low-cost financial literacy classes.

- Online Financial Courses: Platforms like Dave Ramsey's Financial Peace University, Mint, and the National Endowment for Financial Education provide online classes or tools to help with budgeting and financial planning.

- Government and Employer Programs: Some state governments or employers offer financial education workshops or webinars, which may include tax planning, debt relief, and retirement savings advice.

Personal Growth and Development Opportunities

1. Developing a Growth Mindset

- What Is a Growth Mindset?: A growth mindset is the belief that you can develop your abilities and intelligence through hard work, perseverance, and learning. Cultivating this mindset can help you overcome challenges and see setbacks as opportunities for growth.

- Self-Improvement Workshops: Personal development classes often focus on building confidence, overcoming limiting beliefs, and setting long-term goals. These workshops empower you to take control of your future and make positive changes in your life.

2. Self-Discovery and Emotional Wellness

- Mindfulness and Meditation: Workshops that teach mindfulness and meditation can improve your emotional well-being by helping you manage stress, reduce anxiety, and increase your sense of inner peace.

- Personal Empowerment: Personal development programs focus on building self-esteem, assertiveness, and decision-making skills, which are essential for personal growth and successful parenting.

3. Where to Find Personal Growth Classes

- Online Learning Platforms: Websites like Mindvalley, Udemy, or Insight Timer offer courses in personal development, emotional intelligence, and mindfulness.

- Local Community Programs: Check for local workshops on topics like self-help, personal empowerment, or mindfulness offered by nonprofits, community centers, or adult education programs.

- Books and Podcasts: Books like *The Power of Now* by Eckhart Tolle or *Atomic Habits* by James Clear, as well as podcasts like *The Life Coach School Podcast*, can provide inspiration and practical advice for self-growth.

4. Building Long-Term Goals and Vision

- Career Development: Workshops or courses on career development, resume building, and job searching can help you pursue personal and professional growth, especially if you are balancing work and family life.

- Health and Wellness: Personal growth is also about physical health. Many wellness programs focus on how to integrate exercise, nutrition, and mental health strategies to improve overall well-being.

Final Thoughts on Parenting and Personal Development Classes

Investing in parenting, financial literacy, and personal development classes can provide you with the tools and skills needed to build a fulfilling life for yourself and your family. The knowledge gained from these workshops helps you navigate the complexities of parenting while fostering personal growth, financial stability, and emotional well-being.

Remember, every step you take toward learning and growing builds a strong foundation for a brighter future. Whether you're enhancing your parenting skills, strengthening your financial literacy, or pursuing personal growth, these opportunities empower you to lead a life filled with purpose and resilience.

20. Common Concerns and Answers

Facing pregnancy, parenting, or adoption can bring up many questions, and it's completely normal to seek clarity on various aspects of these experiences. This chapter answers some of the most frequently asked questions related to pregnancy health, parenting in the first year, and adoption. By addressing common concerns, we aim to provide you with the knowledge, reassurance, and support you need as you navigate these life-changing events.

Pregnancy FAQs: Health, Support, and Logistics

1. **How do I know if I'm pregnant?**

   - **Answer: Common early pregnancy signs include a missed period, nausea, fatigue, sore breasts, and frequent urination. The best way to confirm is to take a home pregnancy test and follow up with a healthcare provider for a blood test or ultrasound.**

2. **What kind of prenatal care do I need?**

   - **Answer: Regular prenatal check-ups are essential to monitor your health and the development of your baby. These visits typically include blood tests, urine tests, ultrasounds, and assessments of your blood pressure and weight. It's also a time to discuss any questions or concerns with your healthcare provider.**

3. Can I continue working during pregnancy?

   - Answer: Most women can continue working during pregnancy, but it depends on your health, job, and the demands of your role. If you have a physically demanding job or experience complications, you may need to adjust your workload or take time off. Always consult your doctor about any concerns you may have.

4. What if I don't have health insurance or can't afford prenatal care?

   - Answer: There are several options available for women without health insurance, including Medicaid (for low-income women), federally qualified health centers (FQHCs), and charitable organizations that provide free or low-cost care. Don't hesitate to reach out to community resources for assistance.

5. What should I do if I experience unusual symptoms like heavy bleeding or severe pain?

   - Answer: It's important to contact your healthcare provider immediately if you experience symptoms like heavy bleeding, severe abdominal pain, dizziness, or fainting. These could be signs of complications that require medical attention.

6. What kind of emotional support will I need during pregnancy?

   - Answer: Pregnancy can bring a wide range of emotions. It's normal to feel excited, anxious, or even overwhelmed. Consider joining a support group, seeking counseling, or talking to trusted friends or family members. Mental health is just as important as physical health during pregnancy.

Parenting FAQs: Planning for the First Year

1. **What should I expect during the first year of parenting?**

   - **Answer: The first year is a time of rapid growth for both you and your baby. You will face challenges like sleep deprivation, learning to breastfeed or bottle-feed, dealing with teething, and adjusting to your new role. However, it's also a time filled with joy as you bond with your baby and watch them reach important milestones.**

2. **How do I manage sleep during the first year?**

   - **Answer: Sleep can be one of the biggest challenges for new parents. Babies often wake frequently during the night, and establishing a consistent sleep routine can help. Consider co-sleeping (if safe) or creating a separate sleep space for your baby. It's also important for parents to rest whenever possible, even if it means taking naps during the day.**

3. **What are the best ways to bond with my baby?**

   - **Answer: Bonding can happen through physical closeness, such as holding, talking, or singing to your baby. Eye contact, skin-to-skin contact, and** responding to your baby's cries help create a secure attachment. Feeding, whether breastfeeding or bottle-feeding, is another opportunity to bond.

4. How can I take care of myself during the first year of parenting?

   - Answer: Self-care is crucial for new parents. Try to get rest when you can, eat nutritious meals, and ask for help from family or friends. Consider setting up a support network of people who can offer emotional or practical assistance, like helping with housework or watching the baby for a while.

5. When should I start planning for childcare?

   - Answer: It's best to start thinking about childcare a few months before you go back to work, if applicable. Research options like daycare centers, in-home care, or family members who can help. Make sure to visit facilities in person, check reviews, and ask for recommendations from other parents.

6. What are the important milestones to look for during the first year?

   - Answer: Some key milestones include smiling at 6-8 weeks, rolling over by 4-6 months, sitting up around 6-9 months, crawling by 8-10 months, and possibly saying their first word by 12 months. Keep in mind that every baby develops at their own pace, and if you have concerns, talk to your pediatrician.

1. What is the adoption process like?

- Answer: The adoption process typically includes several steps: deciding on open or closed adoption, choosing an adoption agency or attorney, preparing for the legal process (including background checks and home studies), and finalizing the adoption in court. Each state may have different procedures, so it's important to work closely with a professional adoption agency or attorney.

2. How do I choose an adoptive family for my child?

- Answer: If you decide on adoption, you may be able to review profiles of prospective adoptive families. You'll want to consider the family's values, lifestyle, and background, as well as the type of relationship you want to have with the child post-adoption (open, semi-open, or closed). Many agencies offer counseling to help you through this process.

3. What emotions should I expect during adoption?

- Answer: The emotional journey of adoption can be complex and is different for every woman. You may feel sadness, grief, relief, hope, or even joy. Many women report that the decision to place a child for adoption is a difficult one but also one that brings peace when they know their child will have the life they deserve. Consider seeking counseling to help manage these feelings and understand the process.

4. Can I change my mind during the adoption process?

- ○ Answer: In most cases, you can change your mind during the adoption process before signing the final legal paperwork. The laws surrounding adoption vary by state, so it's important to understand your rights and speak with an adoption professional throughout the process.

5. How will I feel after the adoption is finalized?

- ○ Answer: After adoption, it's common to experience a mix of emotions, including sadness, relief, and sometimes guilt. Many birth mothers find that having a post-adoption plan, such as staying in contact with the adoptive family, can help provide peace of mind. It's essential to give yourself time to process these feelings and seek support when needed.

Final Thoughts on Common Concerns and Answers

Pregnancy, parenting, and adoption are profound life events, and it's natural to have many questions along the way. By addressing common concerns and seeking out reliable information and support, you can make empowered decisions that align with your values and goals. Remember that there is no one right path—what matters most is finding the support, knowledge, and resources that help you feel confident in your choices.

21. A Message of Hope and Strength

The journey you are on may be filled with challenges, uncertainties, and moments of doubt, but it is also a path of incredible strength, resilience, and transformation. Whether you are facing pregnancy, parenting, adoption, or any other significant life decision, it's essential to remember that you are not alone, and your ability to navigate this journey with courage and grace is within you. This chapter offers a message of hope and strength to encourage you as you move forward with confidence, knowing that every step you take brings you closer to the life you are meant to create.

Remembering You Are Not Alone

1. The Power of Connection

- **It can be easy to feel isolated, especially during times of uncertainty or when facing life's most difficult moments. But know that you are part of a vast community of individuals, families, and professionals who understand your struggles and are ready to offer support.**

- **Whether it's through family, friends, support groups, or community organizations, there are people who want** to help and stand by you every step of the way. Never hesitate to reach out for support when you need it.

2. Shared Strength

- You may not always see the strength in yourself during tough times, but remember that strength isn't just about enduring—it's about finding the courage to ask for help, to keep going even when you feel uncertain, and to embrace your journey.

- The stories of women who have faced similar challenges and emerged stronger are a testament to the power of resilience. You, too, have the inner strength to overcome obstacles, learn, and grow.

3. It's Okay to Seek Support

- Asking for help is not a sign of weakness—it is a sign of strength and self-awareness. Whether you reach out to a counselor, join a support group, or confide in a trusted friend or family member, seeking support allows you to heal, reflect, and move forward with clarity.

4. There is No One Right Path

- Life is not a straight line, and the journey you are on may take unexpected twists and turns. Trust that there is no "perfect" way to navigate your path—each step you take, whether forward or backward, contributes to your growth and understanding.

1. Embrace Your Unique Journey

- Your path is uniquely yours, shaped by your experiences, values, and dreams. While others may have advice or expectations, only you can determine what is best for you. Trust your instincts and allow yourself the freedom to make choices that feel right for you and your family.

- Recognize that you have the wisdom, creativity, and inner strength to create a fulfilling and meaningful life, even if it looks different from what you expected.

2. Take Small Steps Toward Your Goals

- Big changes and challenges can feel overwhelming, but breaking them down into small, manageable steps can make them feel more achievable. Celebrate each small victory along the way, and remember that progress, no matter how slow, is still progress.

- Whether you're taking the first steps toward parenting, preparing for adoption, or building a life after pregnancy, every action you take contributes to a future filled with possibility.

3. Trust in Your Resilience

- Resilience isn't about avoiding challenges—it's about developing the ability to bounce back, learn, and grow from them. Know that the difficulties you face today will contribute to your strength and wisdom tomorrow.

  - Remind yourself that setbacks don't define you—they refine you. Every challenge you overcome, every lesson you learn, adds to your resilience and empowers you to face the future with confidence.

4. Celebrate Your Strengths and Achievements

  - Take a moment to acknowledge all that you have already accomplished. Whether it's making a difficult decision, seeking support, or showing up each day with determination, you are stronger than you realize.

  - Keep a journal of your accomplishments, no matter how small they may seem, as this can serve as a reminder of your strength and perseverance on difficult days.

5. Embody Self-Compassion

  - Be kind to yourself, especially when things don't go as planned. Understand that growth and progress are not linear, and it's okay to have setbacks or moments of self-doubt.

  - Embrace the journey with compassion, patience, and forgiveness. You are doing the best you can, and that is enough.

Final Thoughts on Hope and Strength

No matter where you are on your journey, always remember that you have the power to create a future that reflects your values, dreams, and strength. There will be days when the road feels difficult, but those are the days when your resilience shines brightest. You are not alone in this journey—reach out when you need support, trust in your ability to grow and adapt, and have faith that you are moving toward a future filled with possibility.

With each step, you are building the strength and confidence needed to create a life that is meaningful and fulfilling. Embrace your journey with hope, knowing that you have the courage and resilience to overcome whatever challenges come your way. You are strong, you are capable, and you are not alone. The future is yours to create.

Disclaimer

The information provided in this book is intended for general informational purposes only and is not a substitute for professional advice. While every effort has been made to ensure the accuracy of the content, the author and publisher are not responsible for any errors or omissions, nor for any outcomes resulting from the use of the information provided.

Always seek the advice of your physician, therapist, counselor, or other qualified health provider with any questions you may have regarding pregnancy, parenting, mental health, or other related topics. The content in this book is not intended to diagnose, treat, or provide a substitute for medical or professional care.

The author encourages readers to seek professional help for any serious or ongoing emotional or mental health issues, and to reach out to local support groups, community resources, or licensed professionals for specific guidance and assistance.

This book is for educational purposes only and reflects the experiences and perspectives of the author and contributors. Individual experiences may vary, and each person's situation is unique.

Ending Letter of Encouragement

Dear Reader,

First and foremost, I want to thank you for taking the time to read this book. The fact that you are here, exploring the resources, stories, and strategies shared within these pages, is a testament to your courage and your desire to create a meaningful, empowered future.

I know that the journey you are on may feel overwhelming at times, whether you're navigating pregnancy, parenting, adoption, or personal growth. Life can be filled with challenges, but remember that every step you take, no matter how small, is a step toward a brighter and stronger future. You have within you a wellspring of resilience, wisdom, and strength that will guide you through this journey.

It's okay to feel uncertain, and it's okay to seek support when you need it. You don't have to face anything alone—reach out to those who can help, whether they are professionals, family members, or trusted friends. By asking for help, you show not just vulnerability, but also strength and self-awareness.

As you move forward, hold onto the belief that you are capable of more than you may realize. Every challenge is an opportunity for growth, every setback is a chance to bounce back stronger, and every victory, no matter how small, is worth celebrating.

Know that you are worthy of love, respect, and support. Your dreams, your future, and your well-being matter. Take things one step at a time, trust in your own abilities, and remember that your journey is uniquely yours.

I believe in you. I know that you have the strength, resilience, and courage to build the future you desire. Embrace each day with hope, with confidence, and with the unwavering belief that you are not alone. Your path forward is filled with possibility.

With love and encouragement,

Robert Anderson Love Wins

http://RobertAndersonLoveWins.com